The French Don't Diet Plan

ALSO BY DR. WILL CLOWER

The Fat Fallacy:
The French Diet Secrets to Permanent Weight Loss

The French Don't Diet Plan

10 Simple Steps to Stay Thin for Life

DR. WILL CLOWER

CROWN PUBLISHERS • New York

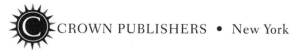

Copyright © 2006 by William Clower, Ph.D.

Published in the United States by Crown Publishers, an imprint of the Crown Publishing Group,
a division of Random House, Inc., New York.
www.crownpublishing.com

Crown is a trademark and the Crown colophon is a registered trademark of Random House, Inc.

Library of Congress Cataloging-in-Publication Data

Clower, William.
    The French don't diet plan : 10 simple steps to stay thin for life / Will Clower.— 1st ed.
        p.   cm.
    Includes bibliographical references and index.
        1. Reducing diets.   2. Cookery, French.   3. Natural foods.   4. Food habits—France.   I. Title.
RM222.2.C527 2006
613.2'5—dc22

2005030998

ISBN-13: 978-0-307-33651-4

ISBN-10: 0-307-33651-4 (alk. paper)

Printed in the United States of America

Design by Helene Berinsky

10 9 8 7 6 5 4 3 2 1

First Edition

To Ben and Grace. 129.

Acknowledgments

I want to thank my family for being supportive during the writing of this work and during the hurly-burly of this funny roller-coaster life.

The best friend I have had in the process of publishing *The French Don't Diet Plan* has been my literary agent, Stephanie Rostan. She's a coach, a sane voice, a go-between, an advocate. In short, she's everything anyone could ever want in a publishing partner. I've said it a hundred times at the bottom of every e-mail, but thank you again, Stephanie.

Stephanie comes to me via the Levine-Greenberg Literary agency—specifically, through Daniel Greenberg, who initially looked at my proposal and decided to move forward on this work. One step back from Daniel is Sumya Ojakli, my longtime marketing advisor and friend who cast the first seed by introducing me to Daniel one year before this work was accepted. The best seeds have a long germination.

My PATH friends and personnel have given me the freedom to write. Kristi Hannon, Rita Hanna, and Amy Young are gifts to work with. I can't believe I'm fortunate enough to have people like them around.

As this book was being written, an exceptional company, Citizens Bank, adopted The PATH for their employees. Their corporate program became a major influence in the creation of this book, as we received critical feedback from their employees on how to best implement the French diet for Americans.

The publicity engine of Crown books, Brian Belfiglio, has been a great support as we've put together plans for making this work visible. Every time I throw an idea his way, and cringe to think I'm bothering him, he writes back right away with his positive and encouraging thoughts. Thanks, Brian.

My editorial contacts at Crown, Katie McHugh and Carrie Thornton, have done a superb job in streamlining prose, refining the sense of my logic, and making sure the voice is consistent. Great job, guys.

Contents

Introduction

*O*n a breezy Saturday afternoon, you stroll along the Saône River that laces across the heart of Lyon, France. Your long-awaited three-week vacation has finally put all your work anxieties behind you. To your left bustles a hive of shoppers at the open-air market, where rows of vegetables are so bright you want to reach out and touch them all. Bags of fragrant spices almost beg you to pinch them.

A little farther and the aroma hits—fresh baked baguettes, still warm and waiting for you to dip their crust into a bowl of olive oil and balsamic vinegar. You'd love to, except that you just finished a lingering love affair with a two-hour lunch: an appetizer of rich fois gras, followed by a tender slice of duck breast with garlic green beans, and a few taut grapes followed by the most luscious cheeses you've ever tasted.

Even after walking for about thirty minutes, you're not short of breath, nor are your legs tired. Your clothes feel looser against your body and, somehow, you've lost a few pounds. You pause at a bench to raise your eyes to meet the stately Fourvière Cathedral across the river, and realize that since arriving, you've eaten whatever you wanted.

You've forgotten your diet.

Despite the ease of the living and the luxury of the food, you've never felt better—or looked better. The only bittersweetness is the fact that you *must soon go home to the harried world of prepackaged quickie foods. And you know that, once you return to that mile-a-minute culture, you'll be right back where you started from. If only you could stay this ener- gized, thin, and healthy. If only you could somehow re-create this atmo- sphere that effortlessly lowers your weight and puts you at peace with your food again.*

After earning my Ph.D. in neurophysiology, I was awarded a position at the Institute of Cognitive Sciences in Lyon, France, to study how our behavioral habits actually change the way the cells in our brains work. I expected to learn a lot about how behavior affects the brain, but I never dreamed that this experience would end up changing my entire thinking about *food*. I saw so many odd things about the French and their diet that just didn't square with my American assumptions about what were—and were not—healthy eating habits.

I found that the French break every one of our dietary rules. And as soon as everyone in my family modeled our eating behavior after theirs, all of us (except the cats) lost weight. My wife, Dottie, dropped that elusive last ten pounds, I shed twenty-five, and my mother went from a size twelve to a six. After these results became so apparent, I found myself awake at four A.M. transcribing my observations, trying to figure out what was going on.

For example, early in our stay, the director of the lab walked us around a typical grocery store. I couldn't get over all the dairy products— rows and rows of cheeses, an entire refrigerated case just for yogurts and crème fraîche. Something felt wrong though, and it took me about three trips to the store to realize what it was.

Where are all the low-fat products?

Each afternoon, I ate lunch in the Neurological Hospital cafeteria with my colleagues. And every day we ate rich, decadent cheeses to finish the meal. The first time they were served, I looked around to see if anyone else hesitated to indulge in food that was so "bad" for you. I asked one of my friends, "Is this cheese high in saturated fat?" To which she replied, "What are you *talking* about?"

Aren't they concerned about eating so much fat?

Just after arriving in Lyon, we stayed at a little hotel in the restaurant district downtown. The September evenings were warm that year and we would've liked the windows open for a draft of cool evening air. But we had to shut them at night because of the ongoing clamor from the cafés outside. Everyone was still eating at the outdoor tables at nine, ten P.M., even midnight. The voices went on, talking and laughing.

Their mealtimes last so long—and they eat so late at night.

We moved from Lyon to settle in nearby Meximieux and, on weekends, my family and I would walk the streets of our little village. People would pass. They'd sit down at outdoor café tables, just talking and sipping coffee or something. One day, as we passed the magazine kiosk, I noticed a cover headline announcing a lead article on *l'obesite Americain*. Then it hit me.

No one's fat here.

The Science Behind the French Paradox

Despite the rich creams, cheeses, butters, and breads, the obesity rate in France is only 11.3 percent of the population (according to a 2005 survey by the London-based International Obesity TaskForce). And all those natural, unaltered dairy products have left these 60 million people with heart disease rates that are a full three times lower than ours. This high rate of heart disease is one of the reasons listed by the World Health Organization to explain our relatively poor life expectancy rating. The WHO released data showing that eight of the top ten countries whose citizens live the longest are from the Mediterranean region, and France is number three. The United States, with all our wonderful health care and prudent nutritional advice, is ranked at number twenty-four.

Somebody somewhere is on the wrong page.

According to the Centers for Disease Control and Prevention, the American obesity epidemic has absolutely ballooned over the past twenty years. The very first assessments, in 1985, reported that no U.S. state had an obesity rate of greater than 20 percent. But by 2003, thirty-one states had obesity rates above 20 percent, and four of them had average rates over 25 percent.

We're only now coming to realize the extent to which our weight problems produce our health problems, such as heart disease and diabetes. Again from the CDC, one American now dies of cardiovascular disease every thirty-four seconds, and this is especially increasing in the fifteen- to thirty-four-year-old category. Diabetes costs consumers more than $132 billion in direct and indirect costs every year.

And while our obesity and all its health consequences were skyrocketing, we were coached to eat low-fat products containing the hydrogenated oils that, it turns out, contribute to heart disease, the high-fructose corn syrup that we now know produces triglycerides, and the diet drinks that turn out to be associated with weight gain.

No wonder we've had such a problem managing our weight and health.

After diet advice has bounced us from low fat to low carb to low sugar to vitamin supplements, we're simply left confused. I speak all over the country and the number-one problem I hear from dieters is that they just don't know what to put in their mouths anymore. Do you remember when margarine was the heart saver? Now it's the heart killer. Nuts used to be bad because of the oils, now they're good because of the oils. Eggs would kill you because of their cholesterol, but now even that's been solidly disproved.

Meanwhile, even though everyone knows that the French way of eating produces low weight, healthy hearts, and longer lives, we still call it a "paradox." Why is that? Of course, the French don't call their own habits paradoxical, but when you look at the most current nutrition science data, the puzzle resolves just as nicely for us as well.

- **The French don't eat processed foods.** A continual string of research results reinforces the commonsense conclusion that our bodies are perfectly constructed to process real food, not synthetic food products. And this makes sense, given our discoveries that faux fats like olestra require an FDA warning label, and faux carbs like aspartame are associated with a closet full of health problems. There are no warning labels on tomatoes, carrots, and onions.

- **The French don't avoid fats.** We've recently discovered that the French were right all along. They've always eaten what we're now calling "good fats," such as those found in olives, nuts, and salmon. Even their daily dairy consumption of yogurts and cheeses is now gathering research support from scientists, who show how these foods may actually promote weight loss.

- **The French don't avoid carbs.** Their carb consumption typically comes from such staples as baguettes, couscous, rice, and potatoes. As we're now finding out in the aftermath of the Atkins revolution, eliminating carbs from your diet may produce short-term weight loss. And yet, without them, the nutritional imbalance causes that ten pounds lost to become twenty pounds regained.

- **The French don't take supplements.** Their culture of getting vitamins from fruits and vegetables, rather than supplement pills, also agrees with lists of studies showing how common synthesized forms of A, E, and C extracted into pills can do more harm than good.

- **The French don't shun wine at lunch and dinner.** We've known for twenty years, but have only recently accepted, that wine is a health food. The French enjoy wine with their meals every day, and it protects their hearts by lowering the bad cholesterol and raising the good cholesterol through its protective polyphenols and resveratrols.

- **The French don't rush through meals.** Is there a more typical French habit than taking your time with the meal? Our physiology responds to this relaxed atmosphere by routing blood to the viscera for optimal digestion. And, because you're eating slowly, your brain gets the neurohormonal message that you're satisfied, so you don't overconsume your food.

The cultural eating habits of the French embrace so much more than our typical straitjacket diets. For example, there are no French eating plans, no diet products to consume at prescribed intervals, no shady ads promising instant weight loss, no cultural obsession around the food group "menace of the moment" (they eat fats, they eat carbs, they eat sugar, they eat proteins). This holistic approach is all the more powerful because it's not a theory at all. It comes as a gift from their history and traditions, centuries old. It's just what they do.

When you break it down piece by piece, it turns out that the French paradox is not so paradoxical at all. The true irony is that we haven't tried the simplest, most obvious solution to our weight and health problems—to apply their approach as a model in our lives. They're thin. They're healthy. We're not.

The Fat Fallacy

In 2001, I published *The Fat Fallacy* to explore these observations of the French diet. It was a new idea at the time to propose that rich wonderful food is *not* the enemy. After *The Fat Fallacy* was released, I received an overwhelming amount of feedback. Many wrote to say how this simple idea had changed their lives, their entire relationship with food, and that they were losing weight on the same chocolates, cheeses, and healthy whole foods that the French eat. Some told me that their hypoglycemia had gone away, and they were freed from having to eat every two hours. Others wrote that their lactose intolerance had disappeared completely. And the best part was when parents let me know how easily they applied this new lifestyle for their kids.

But there was a problem.

We all agree that "if you do what they do, you'll get their results." We all agree that "find success, then copy it" works as a strategy. But translating the principles of *The Fat Fallacy* into practice within the quirky particulars of everyday life here at home presented a challenge. People needed much more structure and guidance in a specific non-dieting "plan." "It makes so much sense," they said, "but *what do I do?*"

We, not the French, are bombarded by television commercials advertising the likes of purple ketchup, low-fat salad dressing, and food products that have more in common with chemistry than biology. Our stores have three times as much faux food as real food, making it difficult to shop for healthy choices. *What do I do?*

The French don't have a lunch period, they have a lunch epoch. We normally have nano-lunches by comparison. One executive colleague informed me that she feels guilty for just taking time to eat. Most of us can't take a two-hour lunch, or even a one-hour lunch. *What do I do?*

Most French cities are living cities, set up for walking, not driving. There are no traditions of being couch potatoes, maximizing screen time, or spending an extra ten minutes sitting in the car, trolling the parking lot for the closest possible parking space. *What do I do?*

They are less committed to squeezing a few more minutes out of the workday than living enjoyable lives. Their relaxed culture gives them a mandatory five weeks of vacation per year. And they're not pushed to perform every second of the day until they collapse into bed. I don't have five weeks of vacation. I'm lucky if I get two! *What do I do?*

The PATH to Healthy Weight Loss

All these concerns raised the need to solve the practical end of this equation. So I created a step-by-step weight loss program as a tool that anyone can use to make the success of the French lifestyle approach work, even in our busy lives. Unlike other support-group environments, our curriculum is taught for credit at the university level, as a corporate wellness program, and is provided for doctors and nurses in a hospital setting.

The PATH to Healthy Weight Loss was created for those who benefit from individual instruction from our staff nutritionists, and *The French Don't Diet Plan* is based on that program.

It is comprised of four key principles:

1. Eat Real Food

The French eat anything they want, as long as it's real. This principle, eat real food, is so intuitive and can be applied anywhere from the family dinner to the office party to the baseball game. Unfortunately, we've become so inundated with what I call faux foods—chemical sugars, synthetic fats, and artificial food products—that now we have to be told what real food really is!

Real foods are those products that are natural, can be found in a standard biology text, and are normally part of the food chain. Sodas never grew from the earth, margarine is an invention, and the dyes, preservatives, and stabilizers that give your food the shelf life of steel-belted radials were never meant for your body.

That's why you, like the PATH participants, can enjoy rich cheeses, fresh breads, chocolates, butters, wines, and so on, because they're real. Your physiology expects nutrition to come from these sources. Is it any surprise then, that invented diet products and chemicals have been repeatedly associated with poor health, not better health? Thus, when you eat real food, you're actually giving your body its nutrition in the very form it needs, whereas diet products work against your body and its natural tendency to be thin and healthy.

2. Learn the HOW of Eating

As a neuroscientist, I was trained to study the relationship between the mind and body, between the brain and behavior. I saw that they are inextricably linked: the brain causes behavior, but your actions change the function of your brain cells in the process. It's a circle. But when I investigated our modern nutrition science advice, I was stunned to find out how little time was spent on training your behavior to change your physiology. Yes, everyone talked about "lifestyle habits," but the lip service was not followed by coaching on how you're supposed to develop those habits.

People on The PATH learn how the Mediterranean people control their portion distortion, chronic consumption, and weight problems in the process—and let me tell you, it's not because of willpower. When you finally let go of the mental headache of counting carbs and calories and fats, and focus on the HOW of eating, your new habits take weight off for you. And, because they're habitual, you don't have to think about your diet anymore, as your new behaviors become trained into your brain in the long term. You can't fall off the wagon; you are the wagon.

3. Reduce Stress-Induced Eating

The French approach to health is so much more broad than our simplistic "calories in, calories out" idea. If someone gets sad and goes into an all-out Breyers binge, they may gain weight because of the calories, but the calories weren't the problem, were they? They were just a symptom of a deeper problem of responding to stress with the consolation of consumption.

Stress-induced eating must be handled or no diet—low fat, low carb, blood type, food combining, you name it—will make any difference at all.

To eat like the French, The PATH teaches the real world techniques for opening the pressure valve, in easy homework assignments that take no more than five to ten minutes. These include meditations, but also techniques to head off the vast array of subconscious saboteurs of your weight and health. Get enough sleep, for example, or you'll gain weight. Learn to laugh every day, love every day, and live every day with a playful spirit, and you'll free your body to release the weight it's holding on to.

4. Being Active Without Exercise

People on The PATH are coached to be active, but to know the difference between activity and exercise. They're shown the strong health benefits of doing activities they enjoy. And the main point of these movements is not the number of calories burned, but how much enjoyment you derive from doing them. That's the only way anyone will be engaged for more than two weeks!

This program shows exactly why exercise must be something you love, not something you're forced to pound out on a treadmill. If you're walking from the cheese counter to the rotisserie chicken stand before ambling over the river to take in the art exhibit, you really are exercising. We've been coached that we must get the heart rate up to x percent of baseline for y number of minutes or it doesn't even count. But it turns out that thirty minutes of daily activity, even if spread over the course of a day, promotes good health just as well.

Can you really eat well, lose weight, and love your food again? People on The PATH program have already gone through the lessons laid out in *The French Don't Diet Plan* and have seen the results. They're eating real foods and developing behavioral habits that keep them in control. They're slowing down, tasting more, and getting the health benefits of chocolate, cheese, wine, and breads *without dieting*. Here are some of the highlights of what we've accomplished so far.

Weight Loss

Allure magazine conducted a "road test" of many popular American diets, including The PATH and Weight Watchers. Individual dieters

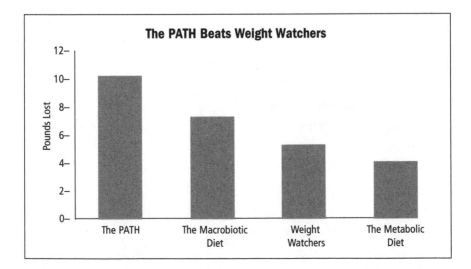

were coached by representatives from each dietary team during a six-week interval. Weights, photographs, and interviews were obtained before and after the trial.

In this six-week head-to-head dietary comparison, The PATH outperformed Weight Watchers and all other national diets. The PATH program produced almost twice the weight loss as Weight Watchers.

Lower Cholesterol

Vail Valley Medical Center is a wonderfully progressive hospital that ran forty-six of their professionals on The PATH curriculum over eight weeks. Participants provided measurements of weight, cholesterol, and behavioral changes before and after. As a group, they not only lost weight, but also achieved significantly lower cholesterol. The average change of 13.3 mg/dL represents a solid decrease in this important marker for heart disease risk.

More important, perhaps, is the fact that this change occurred in a comparatively short period of time, only two weeks after completion of The PATH program. We believe this cholesterol drop results from the consumption of real foods, and the overall decrease in consumption reported by subjects.

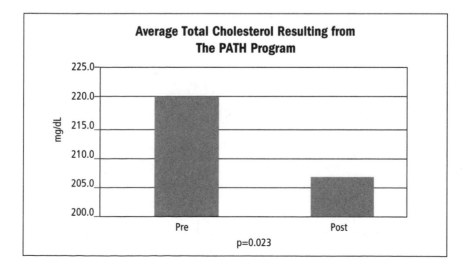

Average Total Cholesterol Resulting from The PATH Program

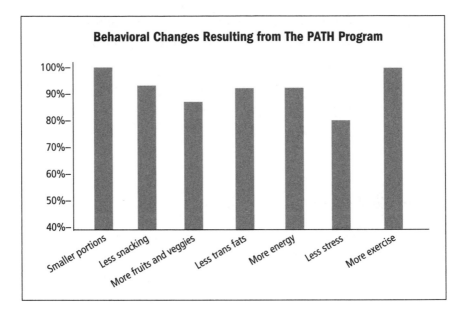

Changing Behaviors for Life

Our corporate wellness clients also reported positive changes in their portion sizes, between-meal snacking, and fruit and vegetable intake. They accomplished this by reinforcing their new behavioral habits of healthy eating.

As research science has found over and over, losing weight is straightforward—keeping weight off is the hard part. But these behavioral changes reported by PATH participants are exactly the kind of results that must be achieved to form the basis for any long-term weight control.

Keeping It Off in the Long Term

In a recent follow-up survey, we asked PATH participants how they were doing over time. They reported how close they were to their target weight, and we plotted that as a function of the number of months they'd been at it. They reported that they were able to maintain their healthy eating habits—and their weight loss—over the long haul.

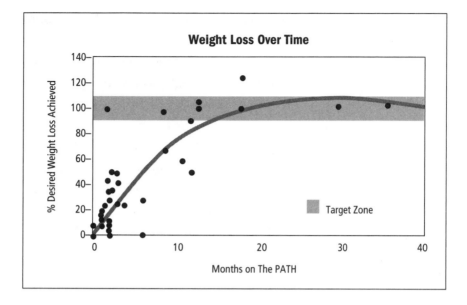

This is the power of The PATH approach embodied in *The French Don't Diet Plan.* You are given the tools to lose weight but, more important, the means to maintain and continue that weight loss for life. In the end, these principles of the French diet end the need for dieting forever, and help you live a life you can love every day.

Why the French Approach Works

We've all heard that diets don't work, and for good reason. Scientific studies suggest that typical dieters regain 80 to 100 percent of any weight they lost within five years. But we keep flogging away at the next fad approach because most people just don't know an alternative. Maybe the solution is to stop trying to make a failed approach work, and stop dieting altogether!

The French don't diet. They do think about their weight—but they don't treat their food as we do—as a list of fats, carbs, and proteins to be eaten in a particular ratio (30 percent of calories by fat as a percentage of total daily intake, based on a two thousand-calories-per-day diet). Who in France orders carbs or fats? No one. They have bread, chicken with vegetables, wine, chocolate, and cheese. When they have weight to lose, micromanaging molecules is the last thing on their minds.

A woman named Pascal lived right across the street from me in little Meximieux. We were chatting about weight issues, and I asked her what French women typically did if they had weight to lose.

The corners of her mouth turned down as her eyebrows arched and she made that *phhhfft*-ing sound. "They don't eat too much again," she said, in her best Frenglish. It was a comical statement, but she was exactly right. In essence, the French change their own behavior so they aren't consistently overeating—that is, "don't eat too much again." That's the point. Losing weight is about behavior, not how some molecule is making one fat. It's exactly why this plan works, and gets straight to the heart of why standard diets don't.

Why Diets Fail

Why do diets fail a full 90 percent of the time? Standard diets tell you exactly what to put in your mouth. Yes, it's true that if you get few enough calories, you're likely to lose weight right away. The starvation diet, like all the rest of them, would work in the short term if you followed the moment-by-moment caloric dictation of what to eat. But most people can't keep up with it every single moment.

You do it for a while, lose a little weight, stop, then your weight comes back.

In other words, diets treat the effects of the problem, not the problem itself. If you blow your nose when you've got a cold, your nose will be dry for a second but then the problem comes right back. Sound familiar? You diet, lose a couple of pounds, but then the problem comes right back. But you cannot live this way. If you cannot follow the dietary dictation and eat leeks or cabbage or fat-free cheese food or carb-free pasta products forever, your weight will just come back, too.

The problem we face is not excess weight—that's just a symptom. So what's the real problem? It's a life out of balance, where volume equals value, where eating is a chore, where the family table is lost, where food is a synthetic invention, and where it's considered normal for children to drink neon sugar water from a thirty-two-ounce Big Gulp cup with a straw in it. There's more going on here than carbs and fats, and the French approach works by going well beyond this starting point.

Fix the real problem, and your weight handles itself.

Diets Don't Work—the Data

A recent study from Tufts University confirmed that none of the major diets (low-fat, low-carb, Weight Watchers, and the Zone) are better than any other at producing weight loss. None of them.

But, as we would predict, the subjects couldn't even stay on the diets for two months (22 percent of them dropped out). By year's end, *a full 50 percent of the low-fat and the low-carb dieters had quit.*

The French Don't Diet Plan

Part One, "What the French Eat," teaches you what delicious foods you can eat so that your food choices are working for you, not against you. Instead of encouraging you to eat new chemicals to outsmart your body, I'll show you why real food is the natural and permanent solution.

Part Two, "How the French Eat," teaches you how to eat well. This is the heart of the lifestyle lessons that make your eating habits permanent. From the fork to the plate to the meal and the restaurant, these habits of healthy eating control portions for you, increase the pleasure of the meal, and remove your fear of food forever.

Finally, Part Three, "Living a Life You Love," handles stress-induced eating with simple daily meditations, as well as practical tips to reduce the chronic consumption caused by stress. Don't forget exercise, but you will notice a big difference in our approach in the very last step.

In the end, this book is your resource. It's your practical daily guide in the store and in the home. So in the back I've added a number of my own recipes, references, and resources to help you establish your new relationship with food. These include flexible, real-world meal plans and a "Rogues Gallery" of faux food ingredients to avoid when you shop.

What You Can Expect

Don't you wonder how some thin people can eat so little? Well, the body is an adaptive miracle and changes based on your eating habits. If you want to eat small like them, if you want to live the French lifestyle of eating, you really can. I'm going to show you how to adapt your physiology and psychology in the right direction. You will train your body to become like those who live the healthy French lifestyle every day.

You are finally going to meet the alternative to dieting, with a new set of healthy habits that become who you are at the fork, plate, and meal. Once you learn these, they'll become habitual, and you'll never have to think about your diet rules again. At that point, your new relationship with food will produce low weight without constant mental effort.

Expect the traditional French eating habits to work just as well at the office, on the road, and even at your yearly Thanksgiving feast. That's the power of this approach: Your new unconscious habits will control your calories for you even when you're not thinking about them.

And just like our mental journey to Lyon at the start of this introduction, you'll feel a freedom and relaxation that you've never had on a diet.

You must have heard the clichés about how the French turn up their noses at bad food. Well, be prepared, because the first adaptation you'll notice in yourself is a change in your taste for high-quality food. People write to say that they simply cannot eat anything other than real foods anymore, because they realize that faux foods taste terrible. When this realization hits, you're finally at the place where you'll never touch chemical faux foods again.

Your cravings for sugar will be the next to go, over a couple of weeks, although some may need longer. And once they do, you'll natu-rally avoid foods with excess sugar added simply because they don't taste as good anymore.

The next change you'll notice will be in your portions at the table, and you'll find that you need far less than you ever thought possible. This change happens when you begin using the behavioral habits that control gobbling. Our very simple changes will reorient your psychol-ogy, too. What looks like just enough begins to normalize. This change will take about a week or so.

Finally, your body will eventually stop needing food between meals. This happens within one to two weeks, much like the decrease you can expect from stress-induced eating. A few basic techniques will re-duce these problems this very night, and you'll see immediate results.

But you won't be eating less, and more healthfully, by marching in lock-step to any calorie counting dietary dictation. You'll be thinner and healthier because you love your food again, because you just can't stomach poor-quality foods, and because you eat all you want to eat— but your body just wants less. You'll do all these things because that's who you've become, and you'll live your new relationship with food every day.

The best part about this approach is that it has been proven to work not only for the French, but for our PATH participants, and in a hospi-tal environment. It's not simply a fad you hope will turn out to be cor-rect one day. It's time we stepped back out of complicated dietary miracle theories and returned to some solid basics of eating for health.

With these tools, you'll be able to apply the habits of healthy eating that produce low weight, healthy hearts, and longer lives for millions of people. And now they'll be yours forever.

PART ONE

⚜ What the French Eat

On the Saône River in Lyon, France, a lively farmers' market sprawls along much of the left bank on most mornings of the week. The first time I came across it, I was astonished at the possibilities beyond our conventional American supermarkets. In this single stretch, vendors sell fifty varieties of mushrooms and more than twenty kinds of olives. The market offered dozens of just-baked breads, hundreds of fragrant cheeses, fresh poultry and game, along with countless herbs, greens, nuts, and legumes. Needless to say, there was not a box of macaroni and cheese or ramen noodles in sight, so I ended up buying fresh green beans, some baby red potatoes, and sliced pork for dinner.

Once I embraced fresh food as normal, I came to realize perhaps the biggest difference between the French diet and our own: They eat real foods, we eat food products. The U.S. Department of Commerce reported that the steady yearly increases in processed food product consumption reached $461 billion by 1993 and is still increasing. The U.S. Department of Agriculture (USDA) reported that the demand for these products is on the rise globally as well.

The problem? Almost all packaged products are laced with an Acme junior chemistry set of preservatives, dyes, thickeners, stabilizers, sweeteners, and acidulants, among other things. The ingredient lists for even the simplest foods, like Healthy Choice ice cream or Wonder Bread, neither of which should have more than five ingredients, consists of rows of unpronounceable microprint. I call these faux foods— and they're directly responsible for sabotaging our weight-loss efforts.

Yes, faux foods are cheaper, because food companies can stamp them out with a shelf life approaching that of plastic. Yes, they're attractive, because these same industries spend $33 billion per year to enroll your favorite basketball star and pop singer to endorse them. Yes, they're tasty, because the chemical sweeteners are synthesized to make it 150 times sweeter than sugar. But despite the advertising claims of added vitamins and minerals, nothing makes those products healthy, and they certainly aren't real foods.

Nevertheless, we eat them. Instead of eggs (cholesterol!) we eat egg substitute. Instead of butter (fat!) we eat margarine. Instead of bread (carbs!) we eat sorbitol-sweetened oxymoronic low-carb pasta. Instead of normal fruits and vegetables for nutrition, we chase junk food with supplement pills. Instead of natural oils (more fat!) our foods have gone through a chemical hydrogenation process.

In this section, I'll show you how a simple return to delicious, ordinary food is the solution for permanent weight loss. The French, not surprisingly, don't suffer our dreadful problems with weight and health— but they don't deprive themselves either. In fact, they're known for the most famously sumptuous diet on the planet and have three times less obesity, three times fewer heart attacks, and they live longer than us— men and women. Think about this: If they can get those results, so can you.

I hear what you're saying already. "I'm not a gourmet French chef. I don't have an outdoor market of wonderful fresh healthy foods in my front yard (and no Saône River either)!" Or maybe you're not sure how you'd ever go without the prepackaged stuff you're used to buying. But I promise that it's easier than you ever imagined it could be to transition from faux foods to real foods, even by shopping in your own local grocery store. Yes, there are a lot of products you'll have to pass up— but this *doesn't* mean you'll be depriving yourself of any favorite meals (including dessert) or the flavors you love. To help you make the transition, we'll walk through every aisle together and show you how simple the switch really is.

But first, and this is the toughest part, you must overcome any thoughts that hold you back. After all, embracing high-calorie foods strikes our diet-centric thinking as just wrong. This is often the first step at my PATH curriculum for healthy weight loss. People invariably ask, "Did you say give up low-fat and fat-free products? Stop counting calories? Forget low-carb diets? Can I really control my weight and still eat delicious foods?"

They're all asking different versions of the same question: "Don't I have to suffer through a hell of deprivation before I'm redeemed with heavenly thin thighs?"

The answer, of course, is no!

Part One takes you on the first three steps toward perhaps the most important part of a lifestyle of better health and smaller pants, the simple difference between what and what not to eat. Don't eat faux-food chemicals. They must be replaced with real foods.

Just as any meaningful change starts at home, Step 1 takes you on an all-out pantry purge. In the process of cleaning out the kitchen, you'll learn the faux-food ingredients that harm your heart and pack on pounds.

Once the fake foods are gone, we're going shopping together in Step 2. We'll stroll the supermarket, aisle by aisle, to find the good amid the bad and the chemically modified ugly.

Because much of the packaged food we're used to is packed with high-fructose corn syrup, an intense sweetener, Step 3 shows how your switch to real foods literally changes what kind of food your body asks for and curbs your sweet tooth for good. Just as your body's need for high food volume will drop over time, your craving for over-sugared foods will evaporate as well. You'll recognize, by taste, just how much sugar fills all kinds of faux foods, and they won't even taste good to you anymore.

In the end, your taste buds will return to normal—and so will your weight. You'll slim down, feel better, and have more energy through the day, effortlessly. And all this starts simply by getting to know real foods again.

Forget Faux Foods

A few weeks before I was scheduled to leave for France, my wife, Dottie, and I attended a neuroscience convention in Washington, D.C. One night, our new French boss-to-be was taking us to dinner to introduce us to his Lyon research team. All dressed up and ready for a lovely meal, we met them on the sidewalk, piled into a cab, and headed over to the restaurant.

As soon as we got in the car, Dottie and I both were immediately distracted by Judith, the team's neuroanatomist. This young French-Portuguese woman was a svelte, flawless, Sophia Loren–type beauty. She spoke with ease and elegance, clearly aware of every nuance of her manner and movements. It was obvious that she was a woman who really took care of herself.

As soon as we reached the restaurant, I became curious to see what such a careful French beauty would eat. I made mental guesses—a sparse green salad with a dot of low-fat dressing, perhaps? A plain chicken breast, hold the potatoes?

I could see her struggling to find something on the menu and understood why only after we got to France, because normally she would order choices like foie gras, a rich duck breast with veggies, followed by a little dessert (a tart or crème brûlée) and some cheese.

At one point, as we chatted and waited for our meals, Judith slowly leaned over the middle of the table to scrutinize the little round packets of nondairy creamer.

"What ees zat?" she asked me, pointedly, as if I were responsible.

"Ah," I responded. Easy question. "That's nondairy creamer."

She frowned. "Yes, but what ees zat?" she said, a bit more emphatically this time. She held one tiny container of the liquid up to the light, clearly disturbed. I started trying to regurgitate my organic chemistry background for a cogent answer when my new boss saved me from my stammer of obscure nomenclature. "It's artificial cream—read the ingredients," he told her. "Americans put it in their coffee."

"No," she breathed. "Een zer coffee?! Zats deesgusting!" Then she warily poked her finger through the remainder of the plastic packets in the bowl, as though she might be bitten by some new lurking threat.

Seizing the moment, I informed her that artificial foods were quite normal here. Hadn't she ever heard of Sweet'n Low? Sugar-free Jell-O? After her near-death experience with the nondairy dairy product, we had her going with outrageous shock and dismay. She'd just never seen the fake foods that I—like all of us—had come to accept as perfectly normal.

Of course, at the time, I thought she was the crazy one. Only a few months later, the tables were turned and my family and I were the ones in culture shock. This time, it was the very lack of artificial foods and quickie prepackaged products around us that was so strange. In fact, we found ourselves forced to buy full-calorie, full-flavor "real" foods simply because there was nothing else to choose from. Our meals always tasted wonderful, but I was sure we'd return from our two years abroad each at least twenty pounds heavier. It just didn't happen. Just a few months into our trip, it became clear that we were breaking every dietary rule in the book and losing weight anyway!

If there are secrets to the French love affair with the meal, or unspoken advice about what's keeping them thin and healthy, the first is their insistence on high-quality natural foods that come from the earth, not a chemical plant. This is so simple, so intuitively correct.

How to Recognize a Faux Food

Avoiding faux foods doesn't sound too hard, until you sift through the parade of products lining our store shelves. How do you know what's healthy and what's not? Take bread, for example. The French eat baguettes every day. But does that make plastic-wrapped spongy "white bread" that lasts for two weeks okay to eat? No! And that begs the question again, how do you know the difference between real bread and fake bread, between real food and faux food?

To sort this out, let's do a thought experiment. Say I took a photograph of a fresh baguette. Our modern technology allows you to see an image that looks exactly like bread. If someone asked you what it was, you could certainly identify it. But would you eat the picture? Of course not. You can see it's not food; it's a photograph.

What if I made a three-dimensional replica from a plastic polymer and painted it so well that it looked exactly like an authentic baguette? Our modern technology can make it look so real that you wouldn't even be able to tell it was fake until you put your hands on it. Would you eat that bread? Would you cut it into pieces, put it in your mouth, and swallow it? Of course not, because you can tell by touch that it's not food. It's a synthetic model.

What if, instead, food chemists made a bread model that simulated the texture of real bread? Our modern technology can replace the harder plastics with synthetic, partially hydrogenated oils.

What if they spritzed the model with odorants so it actually made your mouth water with the homey aroma of freshly baked bread straight from the oven? Our modern technology can produce edible chemicals that easily conjure the smell and taste of wonderful breads.

So the bread now looks like it's not fake, smells like it's not fake, tastes like it's not fake, and even feels like it's not fake. Are you going to eat this bread? Let me tell you, people eat synthetic products designed to appear as though they're not fake every single day!

Some popular diets will tell you it's okay to eat bread, others say to avoid it like the plague. But when it comes to our health, the problem is not with the carbohydrates—it's whether the bread we're eating is actually food or if its nutritional value has been replaced with artificial substitutes.

At one PATH curriculum seminar here in Pennsylvania, a man from the audience spoke to me about his father, who had worked as a food chemist for Heinz many years. He said his dad would come home with little bottles and have his kids try his concoctions. He remembered one bottle of gray gloop in particular. He was told to close his eyes and try it from a teaspoon.

"Ketchup," dismissed the boy. "That's just ketchup."

"Aha!" the father beamed. "But there's not one single tomato in there!"

His father had managed to simulate the taste and feel of tomato ketchup in a chemistry lab. A terrific accomplishment of science, no doubt, but is it food? Of course not.

This is the most stunning, mind-bending fact of our modern technological world. We are allowed, coached, and even encouraged to eat things *that are not food*. Given this tendency, here are some starter rules to remember.

Check the ingredients—they must be natural. And the best foods are ones that don't require labels for you to know what they are!

How to Read Labels

The European Union has tried a couple of times to introduce FDA-style labels with our standard nutritional calculus of the food listed on the back. But they can't get it done because there's just no market for it. No one wants or needs it because they're not agonizing over the grams of protein, fat, and carbohydrates in their foods.

The French don't go to the store to buy grams of this or that. They go to buy food.

That said, here in America, you really should read the labels unless you're absolutely sure of the food source, because of the reasons we've mentioned—that so many normal-looking foods are actually fake. But when you do peruse that periodic table on the back of the box, don't sweat the amount of macromolecules (your healthy eating habits will limit your consumption of them for you!—see Part Two). Rather, look to see whether the ingredients are real; they should have grown from the earth, have had a mama and a daddy, or can be found in a standard biology text.

For example, bread made with flour, salt, water, and yeast is good. That made with thirty-seven unpronounceable ingredients is not— and it makes no difference whatsoever how many carbs, fats, or proteins are in that product. Tons of lab bench chemicals are fat free, and tons more are carb free. But you shouldn't be eating any of them!

I hope you see the point. We've been coached to read labels for the wrong things. By being overly focused on the macromolecules, we've allowed ourselves to eat hydrogenated oils that are harming our hearts and high-fructose corn syrup that helps make us fat. When you read the labels for real foods, you avoid all that because there are no synthetic dyes in an apple or chemical sweeteners in a tomato.

Why Avoid Faux Food?

Never before in human history (until now) have we had to ask the question, What is food? Our biology took care of that for us, through our senses. But now, synthetics can fool our physiology into thinking something's okay to consume, when it's nothing but a cheap imitation, a faux food that undermines your weight and health.

Think about your body like any other machine for just a moment. The synergy between its optimal functioning and its energy source is absolutely vital—the kind of machine, for example, must match the particular fuel it expects. Cars run on gas. Computers run on electricity. And our physiology runs most efficiently on real food. Put a banana in a gas tank and the car won't run. Put gasoline in people and they won't run either.

Real Food for Thought

Why do we have to qualify "food" with the word *real* anyway, as if there's a food out there that's not real?

- All food is real food—so calling it "real" is redundant.
- All inventions are not food.
- So let's just cut the jargon and make life simple: Eat food. And if it ain't food, don't eat it.

You may be twenty-nine years old (and holding . . .), but your body lives at the end of a long genetic thread that's eons old. You exist as part of an ancient living gift whose history trails back far beyond memory. Your physiology *is alive today because of its fuel sources*, which come from the earth.

Strawberry Flavoring

Amyl acetate, amyl butyrate, amyl valerate, anethol, anisyl formate, benzyl acetate, benzyl isobutyrate, butyric acid, cinnamyl isobutyrate, cinnamyl valerate, cognac essential oil, diacetyl, dipropyl keton, ethyl acetate, ethyl amyl ketone, ethyl butyrate, ethyl cinnamate, ethyl heptanoate, ethyl heptylate, ethyl lactate, ethyl methylphenylglycidate, ethyl nitrate, thyl propionate, ethyl valerate, heliotropin, hydroxyphenyl-2-butanone (10 percent solution in alcohol), alpha-ionone, isobutyl anthranilate, isobutyl butyrate, lemon essential oil, maltol, 4-methyl acetophenone, methyl anthranilate, methyl benzoate, methyl cinnamet, methyl heptine carbonate, methyl naphthyl ketone, methyl salicylate, mint essential oil, neroli essential oil, nerolin, neryl isobutyrate, orris butter, phenethyl alcohol, rose, rum ether, gamma undecalactone, vanillin, and solvent.

Look at these ingredients. This is not food.

Over forgotten ages, the food grown here has adapted to us, and we to it. This is a mutual biological understanding, *a relationship*, and it's as strong and established as our species itself. We exist because of this relationship, we thrive because of it, and we compromise our health as soon as we lose sight of it.

Somehow we've moved away from this biological heritage of food in favor of man-made chemicals. We try to fool our taste buds with synthetic imitations, put them in a package, and sell them. But any product of this sort, by definition, cannot be food simply because our physiology has no biological context for inventions. If you need a rule to follow for your best health, don't eat inventions.

If we forget the depth and importance of this most basic synergy, we will undermine the very foundation of our health. Our physiology is not an invention, and its food should not be either. These synthetics have never been alive or a part of the food chain. They've never been a part of our biology or present in the environment before the last biological nanosecond. If you give your body something it has never encountered, that it has no context for or relationship with, you will introduce weight and health problems. You might as well stick a banana in your gas tank.

Need a real world example? High-fructose corn syrup (HFCS) is made to simulate sweeteners like sugar, but your body doesn't recognize it as sugar. That's why your liver, which normally filters toxins, has to process it instead of your insulin response system, leaving you with elevated triglycerides.

The problem we run into is that so many inventions spill from the grocers' shelves that we assume they're normal, nod our heads at the marketing, and eat them anyway: chemical fats, synthetic sugars, drinks made with phosphoric acid and high-fructose corn syrup (aka soda), plasticized fruit sheets, neon ketchup, and snack cakes with the shelf life of motor oil.

Food companies would have you eat butter that never saw a cow and eggs that never saw a chicken. Others would feed you trans fats that the FDA now requires companies disclose on food labels, and the olestra faux fat that wicks vitamins out of your body so that the FDA requires a warning label on any product that contains it. Scads of diet drinks and chemically sugared candy bars and shakes line the shelves.

Now we're finding that these ingested inventions—hydrogenated oils, artificial sweeteners, preservatives, and so on, are linked to cancer (preservatives like BHT) and heart problems (hydrogenated oils). Does this surprise you, really? Who is shocked by the fact that novelties from the chem lab bench create problems in a body that expects normal foods?

Don't eat inventions. We have a hard enough time with our weight and health as it is. Don't create problems!

❧ PEOPLE ON THE PATH

Dear Will,

As long as I can remember, my mom was a fanatic for Coca-Cola. And by the time I went to college I was well entrenched in a four-or-five-Cokes-a-day habit. This lasted until I read about your approach, and I finally gave it up.

In September 2004, my beautiful beach wedding was canceled courtesy of Hurricane Ivan, and we threw together another wedding in four days. After the stress of all that, my new husband and I finally made it to the Keys for our honeymoon, and I felt I had certainly earned a Coke. I was sooo anticipating that first, fizzy sip for breakfast (college habit—horrifying), but when I tasted it, I was sure the can had gone bad. It was awful! Nothing but chemicals and enough sugar to rot my teeth on the spot.

I actually sipped through two cans before I realized that it must have always tasted this way. It was supposed to taste this way! Out came the fresh-squeezed OJ and Perrier (lovely fizz, by the way), and I've never looked back.

By the way, for years I've been on the highest possible dose of prescription acid reducer for acid reflux. After a while on your plan, I take a pill only as needed, if at all.

Thank you so much,
Erin L.

Friend or Faux?

It's time for a fresh start. It's time to clear the corners and cubbies of the old foods that have been keeping you from reaching your goals for so long. You have a chance now for a clean start, like a good thorough spring cleaning for your physiology that will detox your entire system. But before we shop for real food again, we have to get the chemistry set out of the cupboard.

Unfortunately, when you look for real food in your pantry you may find that the most familiar items are the first ones to go! That's because we've been sold these choices for so long that what we automatically think of as "normal" has changed. Normal used to be fruit, now it's Fruit Roll-Ups and fruit-flavored products. Normal used to be Cheddar cheese, now it's Cheddar goldfish. Normal used to be apple turnovers, now it's apple Pop-Tarts. We have become so inundated with food products that we've lost our sense of what real food really is.

But in order to eat clean again, you've got to shed the junk, cleanse your system of faux foods, and find a new, old-fashioned normal again.

Get a large garbage bag (maybe two) and open your cupboards. Read through the ingredient list on every item, looking for the faux-food chemicals that are listed below. Then make a decision—friend or faux? The friends stay, but *the faux has got to go.*

One by one, toss them in the trash. To be sure, at first you'll wince at "wasting" these products, and may consider donating them to a food bank—but then aren't you giving all the faux foods to the people who most need better nutrition anyway? You could ease your conscience by just tossing them into the Dumpster as a commitment to your health, and making a healthy canned or boxed food donation instead. If you return home from the heap and change your mind, don't worry. You can always go back, dig through the banana peels and coffee grounds and find these products again. They'll taste no different than they ever did.

I'll provide very simple guidance on this process (below), so you can approach it in the way that works best for you. First, I've included the worst of the ingredients, so you can pick up each product and scan for the main offenders. If you find one, toss it out. Next, as a backup, I'll list specific examples of the most common chemicals people harbor in their cabinets. If you see any of these, toss them out.

Ingredients: The Faux Has Got to Go

If you need more information on the most popular faux-food ingredients, check our Rogues Gallery in the reference section at the end of this book. But to begin with, just toss out anything found on this short list of chemicals.

What If You're Diabetic?

This condition warrants a close following of your doctor's advice. That said, you still don't have to eat chemicals. Ask your doctor about the insulin-moderating effects of natural foods that contain fiber, fat, or protein, and the way these lower the glycemic index of your carbs.

Examples might include whole-grain bread with tuna salad, pasta with olive oil and garlic, or a potato with a little butter and sour cream.

- Everything with hydrogenated or partially hydrogenated oils, or trans fats
- Everything with additive sugars, such as high-fructose corn syrup, corn syrup solids, polysorbate 80, and all the chemical sweeteners such as aspartame, stevia, Splenda, saccharine, acesulfame K, cyclamate, sorbitol
- Anything with the words *artificial* or *food product* on the label
- All dyes, such as Red No. 40, Yellow No. 6, Blue No. 2
- Sodium nitrite, sodium nitrate
- Potassium bromate
- Propyl gallate

- Olestra
- Mycoprotein
- Monosodium glutamate (MSG)
- Butylated hydroxyanisole (BHA)
- Butylated hydroxytoluene (BHT)

SUSPECT PRODUCTS YOU MAY FIND IN YOUR CUPBOARD
Sodas
Sugar-free products
Powdered pudding
Gravy packets
Canned soups
Crackers
Chips made with hydrogenated oils
Plastic-wrapped snacks
Plastic-wrapped breads
Boxed macaroni and cheese
Boxed potato products
Skillet "helper" dinners
Breakfast cereals

SUSPECT PRODUCTS YOU MAY FIND IN YOUR FRIDGE AND FREEZER
Pie crusts
Microwave dinners
Frozen bagels
Potatoes (fries, tater tots)
Tortillas
Fake dairy products
Low-fat yogurts
Frozen pizza
Frozen oven meals

Write these down and keep them together on a list, and we'll show you how to replace them in the next step, when we walk you through the grocery store.

No Faux Carbs!

Low-carb Crash

What started out with an incredible boom of 930 new low-carb inventions in 2004 became a fading food product line. Recent market analysis in the United States, Australia, and Europe confirm the trend away from these items. The *Sydney Morning Herald* reported that even giant food manufacturers such as Unilever and Nestlé are pulling back due to flagging demand for all low-carb food products.

Here's the dietary irony of the century. The theory behind low-carb diets is that limiting carbs prevents the rapid swings in blood glucose—from spike to crash—that leave you tired and hungry.

Ironically, isn't this exactly what has happened to the low-carb phenomenon itself? The low-carb craze spiked with a surge of super-sweetened promises, and seems to be passing just as rapidly. Just like one of their dreaded high glycemic index foods, the passing low-carb fad has left us tired of diets and hungry for something of substance.

Maybe that's because faux-carb products like low-carb bread, ice cream, and pasta are hopeless oxymorons, or because their chemical sweetener substitutes can cause health problems.

In a recent interview, Donald Hensrud, M.D., a preventive medicine and nutrition specialist at the Mayo Clinic, pointed out that faux-carb alcohols can act as great laxatives—if you're in need of a little diarrhea, cramping, or general digestive discomfort. These faux-carb sugar alcohols come in many forms: sorbitol, xylitol, mannitol, maltitol, lactitol, lycasin, palatinit, and other hydrogenated starches.

Another problem is that faux-carb ingredients are being added to the market so quickly that they haven't been sufficiently vetted by the overworked and understaffed FDA. Initial research shows some to have low carcinogenic activity, but the full story will never be told until the chemical has been in the food supply long enough. Don't wait until then. To be safe, when you're going through the pantry and fridge (diabetics, talk to your doctor), eliminate products that tout themselves as sugar-free. If you're healthy, there's no reason to be eating sugar-free synthetics in Jell-O, puddings, cakes, cookies, and so on. Below are some of the most prominent offenders.

Synthetic Sugar Substitutes: High-Fructose Corn Syrup

Doesn't high-fructose corn syrup sound all earthy and natural? After all, corn and fructose are both natural. But when you read what they have to do to get this product, you realize how contrived it really is. HFCS is produced from refined corn starch through an impenetrable chemical transformation of "liquefaction, saccharification, and refining" that finally results in something called dextrose syrup. Dextrose syrup is then treated with isomerase to morph it into a high-fructose syrup, dextrose monohydrate, and sorbitol. Definitely not quite the same as sugarcane plucked right from the stalk.

HFCS in Your Body

"A high flux of fructose to the liver, the main organ capable of metabolizing this simple carbohydrate, perturbs glucose metabolism and glucose uptake pathways, and leads to a significantly enhanced rate of lipogenesis [fat creation] and triglyceride (TG) synthesis. . . . These metabolic disturbances appear to underlie the induction of insulin resistance commonly observed with high fructose feeding in both humans and animal models" (Basciano, 2005).

SCIENCE-TO-ENGLISH TRANSLATION

HFCS is not cleared from the blood like normal sugar, so the liver has to handle it as it would any other toxin. In the process, it produces triglycerides and fat. Over time, these can lead to weight gain, obesity, and diabetes.

Maybe all that processing is why *your body does not to treat HFCS the same way it does sugar.* The corn refining industry will squawk, but this assertion is simply based on the plain data. Insulin doesn't even recognize HFCS like it does normal sugar. This forces your liver to clean it up just like it does other toxins.

If that weren't bad enough, your liver processes this 100 percent fat-free ingredient by actually *producing* fat and triglycerides—the very things you were trying to minimize! Concludes Stephanie Davail in a 2005 study, "The digestion, absorption, and metabolism of fructose . . . favors de novo lipogenesis [fat creation]. . . . In mammals, fructose is known to be able to raise plasma triacylglycerol concentrations significantly; consequently, this may induce obesity."

So, when reading the labels on your food boxes, eliminate everything with HFCS (if it's in there, you'll likely spot it in the first three ingredients).

Synthetic Sugar Substitutes: Artificial Sweeteners

Aren't those little pastel packets pretty? On most restaurant tables you can find the light pink, powder blue, sunny yellow, and wedding-mint green doses of fake sugars for you to choose from. But none of them are food.

McNeil Nutritionals, a unit of Johnson & Johnson that markets Splenda (also known as sucralose, invented in Britain and developed by Johnson & Johnson), was sued by the Sugar Association in federal court in Los Angeles for their advertising slogan. You've heard it: "Made from sugar so it tastes like sugar." This is worded to make the consumer think it's not fake, when in fact their chemical processing turns it into a chlorocarbon compound that is certainly not found in nature. It used to be sugar but, after their chemical processing, are you still going to eat that?

The problem is that you can find data on Splenda's safety that are positive *and* negative. Even the studies that show no problems at all with eating it simply may not have asked the question in the right way, or tested for the right condition. The drug Vioxx, for example, was tested for arthritis pain but no one thought to test it for heart attack and stroke. The diet drug combination phen-fen may have produced heart valve problems because of the interaction effect between the two drugs—so they are potentially dangerous only when used in combination.

This kind of research ambiguity happens all the time, and drives home the bottom line: If it's been in the food chain for several decades and everyone seems to be fine, you can trust it. Otherwise, you become the little white lab animals for the next new chemical. How else could they possibly figure out things such as the fact that margarine damages your heart (that took forty years) or thalidomide harms women's reproductive systems after the second generation (that took more than twenty years)?

Mixed results for the new chemical sweetener stevia has left the World Health Organization unconvinced of its safety. It seems like stevia should be fine because it's extracted from the leaves of the South American *Stevia rebaudiana* plant. But even with these natural origins, its importation has been banned in Britain, canned in Canada, and flunked by the FDA—the European Union didn't approve it either (Ephedra, also an "all-natural herb" supplement pill taken for weight loss, was banned because it caused higher risks of heart palpitations, tremors, and insomnia, according to the National Institutes of Health).

Most Americans don't know that the chemical aspartame, found in hundreds of products from Jell-O to diet sodas, has been embroiled in controversy since its FDA approval was revoked for hiding the health damage it caused in experimental animals that ate it. It was reapproved in 1981 after Reagan took office. (At the time, Donald Rumsfeld was CEO of the company that made aspartame, and was on Reagan's transition team.)

Even now, no chemical additive evokes more powerful emotions on both sides of the debate. When you read about aspartame, you'll hear plenty of evidence for and against it. The chemical company points to studies saying aspartame is as good as mother's milk; other researchers, such as Dr. John Olney of the Washington University School of Medicine, point to their studies showing that it kills brain cells in the hypothalamus (the area that helps control weight regulation!), and a Canadian group showed that aspartame exacerbates the brain wave pattern of children with absence epilepsy (see *aspartame* in Appendix II: A Rogue's Gallery of Faux-Food Additives).

Consumers are rightfully concerned about what happens when aspartame gets warmer than only 87°F—it degrades into formaldehyde, methanol, and formic acid, all of which can be toxic on their own. The company that profits from your purchase of aspartame says not to worry about it—and they've sponsored plenty of research to make their point.

I'm not here to settle this squabble, only to say that the safest approach to health is to be conservative and eat real food. Remember, all businesses will say the same thing, just like a telephone recording: "There's no evidence our product causes harm." But *the absence of evidence is NOT evidence of absence*. I could pour together some brand new combination of motor oil and Windex in my basement and the same statement—"There's no evidence that this particular product causes harm"—would hold true. And if some study does come along that implicates harm in any given product, it's a simple matter to dispute some aspect of its methods and materials so you can still say, "There's no evidence . . ."

For your weight and health, be conservative. Eat food that you know is healthy for you, not an invention that you hope might not be bad for you!

No Faux Fats!

For decades, the low-fat dogma was the only answer to weight and health questions. But not only did the theory fail, people couldn't make it work in their lives—it failed the practical test. Now, instead of being instructed to severely cut fat grams from our diets, we're coached on the difference between good fats and bad fats. Giving up eggs, it turned out, was a bad idea. Giving up nuts, it turned out, was a bad idea. Giving up salmon, it turned out, was a bad idea.

Science may double back on itself like this, but doesn't it always come back to something suspiciously close to the French approach? This culture has always intuitively known about good fats and bad fats.

And we're just now getting over our low-fat flirtations to come back around to their conclusions. We've circled the block; they've never moved.

A big reason "low-fat" eating failed to improve our health was that the decrease in fat caused an increase in sugar consumption. If you're selling cookies, and you've taken the fat out, you still have to make the cookies taste good, and cheaply, too. So what do you put in them? More sugars, such as high-fructose corn syrup!

Another reason is that the faux fats, or "trans fats," found in many low-fat products can be disastrous for your heart. Research published in the *American Heart Association Journal* showed that trans fats raise your LDL, or "bad," cholesterol, lower your HDL, or "good," cholesterol, and stiffen your artery walls so they can't respond to pressure changes as well. Because of results like these, the Harvard School of Public Health has estimated that trans fats could be causing as many as thirty thousand premature heart disease deaths every single year. Yes, this chemical increases a Twinkie's shelf life, but it decreases your shelf life! Despite the link between trans fats and heart disease, the FDA recently estimated that more than 40 percent of all food products still contain them.

Some products are simply labeled "fat-free" for sales purposes. Many candies, from Peppermint Patties to Twizzlers, are advertised, perversely, as "low-fat" foods (as if this makes eating candy a healthy choice for dinner). Coca-Cola, in this sense, would be a low-fat food, as would a bucket full of corn syrup. These deceptive ads play on one of the most entrenched of our dietary assumptions—the notion that you'll be thin and healthy if you eat low-fat products.

Toss them all, except for the real foods that can also advertise themselves as low fat: buttermilk (which is low fat by definition), molasses, and vegetables.

No Faux Drinks!

All sodas are faux. I know it's hard, but if you want to lose your weight and regain your health, you've got to break this habit. In fact, avoiding soda—*even diet soda*—is one of the simplest things you can do to take back your health and let go of that weight. For example, Sharon Fowler at the University of Texas Health Science Center recently reported that the more diet sodas you drink, the greater your chances of being overweight! There was a "41 percent increase in the risk of being overweight for every can or bottle of diet soft drink a person consumes each day," Fowler says.

In addition to causing weight gain, the ingredients can contribute to osteoporosis. One proposed cause for this is that phosphoric acid siphons calcium from your system. Every cell in your body needs calcium, so if soda robs it from you, your body robs it from your bones.

No Bones About It

"In 5,398 college alumnae, 2,622 former college athletes and 2,776 nonathletes, . . . a statistically significant association between nonalcoholic carbonated beverage consumption and bone fractures" (from the Harvard Center for Population Studies).

SCIENCE-TO-ENGLISH TRANSLATION

Drink more carbonated beverages, get more bone fractures.

What happens when your bones run short of calcium? You can get fractures, breaks, and osteoporosis, and this happens in the young as well as the adult population. In 2003, the *Journal of Bone and Mineral Research* reported that carbonated soft drinks and bone density are essentially buckets in a well—when one goes up, the other goes down. The researchers found it didn't matter whether this was the diet or regular variety.

No Faux Veggies (aka Supplements)!

I was once interviewed on a radio station where the host playfully listed all the reasons some people dislike the French so much. "But the main reason," he ranted, winding up for his punch line, "is that they eat all that food we wish we could eat, and it still doesn't make them fat . . . and they do it on purpose!"

His comments reminded me of Dr. Paul Rozin's work on the psychology of food across cultures—particularly between French and American perspectives. In one telling experiment, Rozin compared American and French attitudes toward consuming supplements versus foods. He asked a number of people whether they would rather take a pill to satisfy their nutrient needs, or just eat food. The largest contrast in the entire study was between French males (who could not imagine such a thing) and American females (who were largely okay with the idea).

This finding, of course, reflects our love/hate, loathing/craving relationship with food that reduces the act of eating to a necessary evil of molecule-input for our bodily machines. For too many of us, eating is not about joy and discovery and flavor and celebration, but a chore and an errand. Why else would we rather have the "red wine pill" instead of a glass of wine? Yes, they're actually making a "resveratrol" pill now to substitute for red wine!

The French don't pop supplement pills every day. These healthy people don't need to because they're getting their nutrition from food. "But what's the harm," purr the marketers, "in taking one vitamin pill? It's just like having a little in reserve." I'll go over the science below, but there's a principle you need to hold on to and remember.

Pills are for sick people.

If you have an illness, you need medicine. If your physiology is normal, you should get your nutrition from the same source your body has always relied on . . . food. So if you're sick, please take a pill for your condition. But you can overdo anything, including vitamin supplementation, which can lead to serious health problems. If you're basically healthy, get your nutrient needs filled by food.

Hippocrates, the Father of Medicine before Big Pharma, told us that food is your medicine. Whatever happened to that idea?

An Apple a Day, Not a Pill a Day

"It is sensible and harmless to take a multivitamin and mineral pill for peo-ple in risk groups, e.g., people eating very little or who have an unbalanced diet (children, old people, patients).

"Except for these groups it is poorly documented that vitamins and minerals in large doses have a preventive or therapeutic potential. The largest health potential lies in a healthy diet" (Meltzer, 2004).

Supplements Gone Wrong

A few years ago, the U.K. food watchdog group the Food Standards Agency pointed out the needless use of vitamin supplements: "Most people . . . do not need to take vitamins or dietary supplements be-cause many foods are naturally high in vitamins or have been fortified with them." And in 2003, an article in the *British Medical Journal* pointed out that vitamins can even be harmful.

Sir John Krebs, former chairman of the agency, was quoted as say-ing, "While in most cases you can get all the nutrients you need from a balanced diet, many people choose to take supplements. But taking some high dose supplements over a longer period of time could be harmful."

Here are some key examples, but if you're concerned about getting the best nutrition, be sure to look up the list of food sources for vita-mins and minerals in our reference section.

Vitamin A, Carotene, and Cancer

Beta-carotene is a building block of vitamin A and is found in many green and yellow fruits and veggies. In the context of foods, it has been found to fight diseases from breast cancer to the recurrence of polyps. Yet supplements of synthetic beta-carotene do not. In the massive Women's Health Study sponsored by the NIH, 19,939 women took beta-carotene supplements and 19,937 women took a placebo. Of the women who took beta-carotene, 378 got cancer (369 for placebo takers), 42 had heart attacks (50 for placebo takers), and 14 had other cardiovascular-related deaths (12 for the placebo takers).

In other words, beta-carotene does not work as a cancer fighter when you abstract it into a pill. In fact, for smokers, it can even increase the risk of lung cancer! In two exhaustive studies by the National Cancer Institute with more than fifty thousand participants (the Beta-Carotene Cancer Prevention Study and the Carotene and Retinol Efficacy Trial), beta-carotene supplements increased the likelihood of lung cancer in smokers by about 15 percent in one case and 28 percent in the other.

That's a lot of work to confirm a simple message: Get your carotenes from food.

Vitamin C and Cardiovascular Disease

Vitamin C is an important water-soluble vitamin also known as ascorbic acid, and can be found in a variety of fruits and vegetables (we can't make our own vitamin C, so it must come from food sources). Citrus fruits, tomatoes, broccoli, and all varieties of peppers contain an absolute trove of this potent antioxidant.

Because of these healthful properties, vitamin C supplements were assumed to aid in the prevention of cardiovascular disease. But the U.S. Preventive Services Task Force recently reported that they simply couldn't recommend these supplements. Another research group found the exact same nonresult—vitamin C supplements did not improve the blood markers for heart disease.

And listen to this. Aaron Folsum, in a 2004 study, found that a high vitamin C intake from supplements is associated with an increased risk of cardiovascular disease mortality in postmenopausal women with diabetes. It's not a problem with oranges, or with broccoli and peppers, but with concentrated molecules abstracted and eaten as pills every day.

Vitamin E, Stroke, and Heart Disease

Vitamin E is a fat-soluble vitamin found in nuts such as almonds, peanuts, and hazelnuts, as well as in spinach and broccoli. These foods have been repeatedly associated with a reduced risk of stroke.

But a 2005 study published in the *Journal of the American Medical Association* from the Heart Outcomes Prevention Evaluation (HOPE) trial of nearly ten thousand people concluded that there is no benefit at all from vitamin E supplementation. In fact, "patients in the vitamin E group had a higher risk of heart failure . . . and hospitalization for heart failure." Maybe that's because a pill of four hundred international units (IU) of vitamin E should give you more than twelve times the recommended daily allowance (RDA), but actually only changes its blood levels by 3 percent. Between your mouth and your bloodstream, something else is happening.

As noted Harvard Medical School researcher Michael Gaziano pointed out in 2004, "Currently, the American Heart Association maintains that there are insufficient efficacy data from completed randomized trials to justify population-wide recommendations for use of vitamin E supplements in disease prevention."

Calcium and Weight Control

This is a new angle for the dairy industry. It used to be "Milk, it does the body good." Now it's all about the link between food sources of calcium and weight loss. Researchers are now finding that a diet high in calcium also may help prevent the weight regain and yo-yoing we're so familiar with.

What do the French finish their meals with? Cheese after lunch, cheese after dinner. They eat yogurt for breakfast, too. Now another piece of the French paradox makes sense!

But it's not about the calcium alone—the health benefits of these dairy foods do not materialize when the active ingredient is abstracted into a pill. In one exhaustive review, seventeen studies were assessed and only one of them showed any effect of weight loss with the use of calcium supplements.

As stated by Dr. Zemel, the lead author of many of these studies: "These findings are further supported by . . . data demonstrating a profound reduction in the odds of being obese associated with increasing dietary calcium intake. Notably, dairy sources of calcium exert a significantly greater anti-obesity effect than supplemental sources in each of these studies."

Calcium and Kidney Stones

I was floored at this one. Dr. Walter Willett and colleagues at the Harvard School of Public Health analyzed the data from the massive Nurses' Health Study to see the effect of calcium supplements on bone health. But do you know what they found?

Calcium consumed in food helps prevent kidney stones, but taking supplements actually *increases* one's risk! I never saw that published study on the supplement commercials, but here's what Dr. Gary Curhan at Boston's Brigham and Women's Hospital concluded in the *Annals of Internal Medicine:* "High intake of dietary calcium appears to decrease risk for symptomatic kidney stones, whereas intake of supplemental calcium may increase risk."

Debunking the Supplement Myth

Vitamin companies want you to believe you're prone to nutritional deficiencies, even if you eat bushels of fruits and vegetables all day, every day. That's because, the thinking goes, our conventional methods of agriculture produce crops that are nutritionally vacuous. They look nice, but contain little of value inside. That's the rationale, anyway, and it's amazing to me how many people believe they should exchange food for pills. But think for just a second about why exactly that is.

Why do we recommend an aspirin to prevent heart disease, but not a glass of wine? Why do doctors overwhelmingly prescribe Ritalin to our children for behavioral problems, when behavioral therapy is a viable option? Why do doctors prescribe cholesterol-lowering drugs, even though a modified diet and exercise produce the same desired effects? We know drugs can be lifesavers and are critically important to health, but why do we treat them as the first resort instead of the last?

We do all these things because there's a steady demand. When it comes to weight loss, our pill culture has Alzheimer's disease. We don't seem to remember suffering through the trauma of phen-fen heart valve problems and ephedra-related deaths. All this has happened and much more, and yet we keep coming back for more pills to outsmart our bodies—for the promise of a quick-fix miracle.

We also do all these things because there's a steady supply. I coach my kids—and I'm sure you do, too—to *please* not believe the drug-pusher "friend" who tells them how great they'll feel once they try pot, or meth, or crack, or cocaine. What he says is not true. He's selling something. But we need to be aware that the same motivation is true for the beautiful ads for legal drugs: the television commercials sparkling with playful actors with perfect white teeth and the magazine ads showing happy people living the kind of life they know you want.

Okay, marketers are certainly not crack dealers, but they are all selling something, trying to find the best possible way to present their pills so you'll fund their enterprise. That's why you can't believe even what legitimate drug companies say just because they say it. It's their job to find out what you need to hear, and then say it to you. In fact, if they say it, their conflict of interest gives you far more reason to doubt than to believe.

Are Our Veggies Nutritionally Vacuous?

After reviewing studies comparing foods grown organically (without pesticides and fertilizers) to those grown using conventional modern methods, the results are mixed—evidence can be found to support either side. Nothing's ever easy, is it?

First, there really are differences in the nutrient content of organically grown produce, as compared to the mass-produced varieties. Here are the examples, and please refer to the original articles found in the selected bibliography (Nutrition and Our Food Sources).

1. Organic tomatoes have slightly more vitamin C, carotenoids, and polyphenols.
2. Organic plums have more antioxidant vitamin C, vitamin E, beta-carotene, total polyphenols, phenolic acids, and flavonols.

3. Organic leafy veggies and potatoes have more vitamin C.

4. And another study didn't say what veggies they measured, only that organic produce contained significantly more vitamin C, iron, magnesium, and phosphorus and significantly fewer nitrates than conventional crops.

That's why people buy foods at farmers' markets, because they are more healthful. The problem is that the studies to date haven't shown nutrient differences in the bloodstream. For example, Dr. Caris-Veyrat and his research team from Avignon, France, tested subjects who ate either organic tomatoes or conventional tomatoes for three solid weeks, to see if they could detect changes in their blood levels of the antioxidants vitamin C and lycopene. However, there were no differences between the two groups at all.

Thus, the nutritional difference between organic and conventional foods is there, but it's small—and it certainly doesn't justify the claims that you should take vitamin supplements. Actually, the bigger issue may not be what's missing from conventional produce (the nutrients) but what's added to them (the residue levels of pesticides still in the produce that you and your kids are eating).

My guess is that conventional fruits and veggies are only slightly less healthful, but may be a great deal more harmful, and popping supplement pills isn't going to help with that. Practically speaking, you have to do the best you can with the local grocery stores where you shop. Buy organic whenever possible. If you can't, get conventional fruits and veggies so you don't have to resort to faux foods.

Troubleshooting Faux Foods

So how did cleaning out your kitchen go? Below are some of the most common problems people run into when getting rid of faux-food products.

✤ *Problem: What am I going to eat now?*
   Solution: Get the right resources.

Without frozen pizza and microwave popcorn, how can you survive?!

Most people want to eat healthfully, but just don't know what to do. The first solution is to get a cookbook that makes it super simple. We have more than fifty real foods recipes in the back of this book, and these are just things I throw together at my house, in the middle of my crazy life. Other alternatives include great cookbooks for everyday meals in thirty minutes or less from Mark Bittman and Rachael Ray.

Decent grocery stores will have prepared meats and sides near their deli section made from great materials, all marinated and spiced and ready for you to just cart them home and stick them in the oven! These make delicious quickie dinners, and they normally have a wide variety to choose from. So you can have sushi one night, crab-stuffed salmon another, and Cajun pork chops the next.

❦ *Problem: What am I going to drink now?*
Solution: Keep it simple.

We've become so inured to the presence of soda in our lives that many people honestly don't know what the alternatives are (read more about these in Step 6).

Water is the drink of choice. Pour a small glass of water with dinner, even if you don't plan on drinking it—you'll end up having some, getting used to it, and soon you'll be asking for it specifically, even when you go out to eat! Throw a cut lemon wedge in for a little added tang.

Tea and milk are great options, as are modest levels of beer and wine. Juice is okay when the glass is kept small, but you could also spruce it up a bit with carbonated water—especially if you miss your fizzy drink. Coffee in moderation (one to three cups per day) helps stabilizes insulin levels.

❦ *Problem: What if I don't have enough time to cook?*
Solution: Use simple timesaving techniques.

First, you have to remember the difference between a cook and a chef. A chef is a trained professional who can spend hours and hours laboring over a dish to perfect the precise flavors. Great. But no one has time for this in the real world, and if you think you have to be a chef to eat well, you're just going to resort to prepackaged boxes of preservative-laced food. So you have to think like a cook, one who can get a great meal on the table in just about thirty minutes.

The broiler or grill is your friend. Pork chops, fish fillets, and chicken cutlets need just a little seasoning and they're done in fifteen minutes flat. Start with olive oil, salt, and pepper. Branch out from there later on, but you can just begin with those to make just about anything taste good.

Don't be afraid of the frying pan. Just sauté (read, fry) your veggies in a healthy oil like extra-virgin olive oil, salt, and pepper, and they're done in ten minutes. Green beans are great sautéed, as are the combination of onions and mushrooms. Very simple.

✤ *Problem: What if I have concerns about carbs and blood sugar?*
Solution: Balance carbs with a little fat, fiber, or protein.

If you have insulin instabilities, you might be worried about maintaining your glucose levels between meals. These fears are fed by the most recent dietary fad, which coaches you to eat throughout the day. As always, please consult your doctor related to any medical conditions.

But from my point of view, your first step is to stay away from overt sugar sources, such as regular sodas or overly sugared food products. Beyond this obvious starting point, the key to keeping your insulin on an even keel is to eat small and eat with balance. That is, have your carbs with a little fat, fiber, or protein: a piece of whole-grain bread with a little peanut butter is fantastic, as are peaches with a little cream, macaroni with a little cheese, and so on. When you eat with balance, your insulin and blood sugar stay balanced as well.

Don't Forget, Don't Diet

Most run-of-the-mill diets have you do a start-up detox phase. In this portion of each plan, you're told to cleanse your system of the toxins that have built up by eating whatever novel foods the diet says are bad for you (carbs, fats, you name it). This stage is short because the foods you are allowed to eat are practically impossible to eat for very long.

But when you simply jettison the chemistry cabinet in favor of real foods, your body is released to clear any toxins quite naturally. Your own physiology knows what to do, and how to maintain itself with optimal health when you simply give it real food. This is such an easy rule to remember, and will become completely intuitive after the first few delicious weeks.

Now that you're resolved to avoid eating inventions, the next step—choosing real foods—will give your body back its health.

CHEAT SHEET: EATING FAUX FOOD–FREE

Get out the junk. Give your body the real food it's asking for and you'll provide it with everything it needs for optimal weight, a healthy heart, and longer life.

Finding the Faux
- Eliminate all low-carb, faux-carb food products, such as those that contain sorbitol and aspartame.
- Eliminate all low-fat, faux-fat food products, such as those that contain hydrogenated oils and olestra.
- Throw out all soda.
- Get your nutrition from your food, not supplements. Pills are for sick people.

The Results You're Looking For
IMMEDIATELY
- You will remember how wonderful natural foods taste.
- You will realize how much more satisfying natural foods are than their faux-food counterparts.

WITHIN TWO WEEKS
- You will find that you have more energy through the day.

WITHIN A MONTH
- You will no longer crave your carbonated soft drinks.
- You will find that you can't go back to old faux-food standards.

HOMEWORK: WHERE TO FIND THE FAUX

1. Clean out your pantry.
2. Clean out your refrigerator.

Use the list of faux ingredients to make sure these chemicals are gone for good.

Choose Fabulous Foods

When you jettison faux foods for their fabulous real food equivalents, you discover a world of flavor you didn't even know was there. Suddenly the joy of eating makes an indelible impact, and you become aware of flavor as you never were before. Loving your food again puts eating and the meal itself back into the context in which it belongs.

For example, in a recent article in *Marie Claire* magazine, an American woman was put on a typical French diet and a French woman on an American diet, and their progress was followed for just two weeks. I was asked to provide the eating rules for each. The short story is that the American who followed the French diet lost weight and the French woman who ate like Americans gained weight. But more interesting was what happened after it was all over.

The American woman, Melanie, had just finished with the French diet of real food every day and was invited to a friend's Super Bowl party. She was ready for the works: chips and salsa, buffalo wings, mini pizzas. As she put it, after piling her plate: "I snag a seat on the couch, bring a salsa-fied chip to my lips . . . and spit it into my napkin. Yuck!

"Wait a minute, I tell myself, this can't be right. I choke down a bite of everything else on my plate before admitting to myself that I don't want this gross food. I want roasted potatoes and vegetables with rosemary and thyme. I want cheese and a loaf of crusty bread. I want to be French forever! I stroll to the kitchen and dump my plate of junk in the trash."

Real foods have the best flavors. When you introduce them back into your life, you realize how wonderful they are and how insipid faux foods actually taste. And you don't have to do anything incredible or heroic in the kitchen as a chef . . . just eat real food.

Staples to Stock

Nonrefrigerated Foods

CANNED FISH
> Salmon
> Sardines
> Tuna

GRAINS
> Couscous
> Granola
> Oats
> Pasta
> Rice

VEGETABLES
> Beans (pinto, white, field peas, chickpeas, green beans)
> Onions (sweet and red)
> Potatoes (yams, new, and other varieties)
> Pumpkin
> Tomatoes

OILS AND VINEGARS
> Extra-virgin olive oil
> 100 percent vegetable oil
> Vinegar (white or red wine, balsamic)
> Walnut oil

BAKING ITEMS

- Baking powder
- Cocoa powder
- Cornstarch
- Flour (all-purpose or whole wheat)
- Herbs / spices
- Sugars (white or brown)
- Pepper
- Salt
- Vanilla extract

SNACKS

- Crackers and chips (nonhydrogenated)
- Dried fruit
- Hummus
- Marinated mushrooms
- Nuts (any variety)
- Olives
- Popcorn kernels
- Salsa

CONDIMENTS

- Capers
- Mustard (spicy or yellow)
- Olive paste
- Pickles
- Real mayonnaise
- Soy sauce
- Sun-dried tomato spread
- Tabasco sauce

Refrigerated Foods

DAIRY

- Butter
- Cheese

Eggs
Milk
Yogurt

DRINKS
Coffee
Beer
Juice (100 percent fruit)
Milk
Tea
Water
Wine

VEGETABLES
No restrictions here

FRUITS
No restrictions here, either

MEATS
Beef (rarely)
Chicken
Deli items (ham, turkey, pepperoni, and so on)
Fish
Pork

Shopping for Real Foods

Years of dieting have conditioned us to hop between food groups, as weight-loss fads have come and gone. After all, how many of you filled your shopping cart with rice cakes and margarine when the low-fat dogma was the end-all answer? How many of you tossed out every potato and banana in your house to purchase bacon, eggs, and cheese when low-carb dieting was the rage? First you were coached to be afraid of fats, then carbs, then bad fats, then bad carbs, and so on. Take them all back!

When you live the French lifestyle you will change your food choices without having to analyze another set of macromolecules. Now when you go to the grocery store, you'll be shopping for food, not molecules. That way (thank heavens), you don't have to mentally deconstruct the biochemistry of your food in the aisles! This lifestyle change releases you from any need for carb, calorie, or fat counters, and replaces them all with nothing more than high-quality foods. This is so refreshingly easy.

Formerly Forbidden Foods, Welcome Back!

If you have been chasing fad diets, you've had to wave a tearful good-bye to some wonderful foods. Now you can bring them back.

- Low-fat people: cheese, butter, ice cream, chocolate, salmon, cream, all nuts
- Low-carb people: rice, bread, potatoes, normal sugar, all fruits, all vegetables, wine, beer

---

So it's time now to return to the sane middle ground and eat real foods again. You can do this, but there are several pitfalls you have to negotiate as you weave your way through the aisles.

First, don't give in to embarrassment, like when your kids writhe about on the floor over your momentary hesitation to buy the chocolate-frosted-sugar-bomb cereals. Don't cure their *epilepsy de sugar bomb* by dropping the dyed corn syrup balls disguised as cereal in the cart. Just keep moving. They'll get over it.

And you've heard this before, but it's important—don't shop hungry because that makes everything look good. I once went camping for five days when I was younger, tromping around with forty pounds on my back. At the end of the day we'd whip out our boxes of dried "starch and spice packet" grossness and boil it in siphoned stream water. It tasted five-star fabulous, and I couldn't get enough. Later, when my body wasn't drunk from fatigue and famine, I tried this particular product again and it was road-kill horrid—the texture, the flavor, all of it. I couldn't believe I had ever been in a situation where I liked it—much less loved it.

So schedule your shopping right after a meal and, if you are taking your kids along, don't even go near the cereal aisle.

Another big help on this excursion: Bring a list. I know, I know, that sounds simple, right? But if you've ever gone to the store without one, you know that you forget the items you were supposed to come home with and buy all kinds of stuff you don't really need. Also, when you make out your list, you can do it with an eye toward the next few meals. Buy only what you need for those immediate dishes: garlic, onion, mushrooms, fish, and so on. And be sure to check our recipes in the back for your dinner tonight, and the ingredients you'll need for them.

Step by Step Shopping from A to Z

Standard grocery stores have the same basic layout. The fresh foods are arranged around the periphery of the store, the freezer aisles are somewhere in the middle, and the impulse candy is stacked up in the checkout line (the nutritional equivalent of the quality reading material it shares space with). Unfortunately, each section of the store has its own shopping challenges for the person who wants to eat real food. You'll need to understand the trade-offs you face, the products that are good for you, and the food products you should avoid altogether.

Carry this guide with you to the store to help with your food choices in every single aisle. After a couple of trips, you'll have it down pat.

A. Fresh Fruits and Vegetables
Virtually every grocery store presents you with the look and feel of good food and good health as you enter it. Banks of open-market style fruit and vegetable bins border your weave through this section. How can you go wrong with fruits and veggies? Well, there are some considerations.

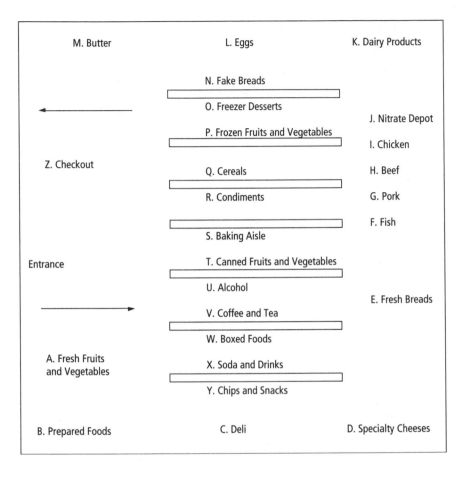

First of all, unless the sign says LOCALLY GROWN, chances are that the fruit was picked green, shipped in from somewhere far away like Latin America, and gassed with ethylene. Ethylene is produced by the combustion of kerosene, and also by ripening fruit itself. They gas the fruit right before it's released into the "fresh from the tree" bins in a process called de-greening.

Everyone asks if they *have* to buy organically grown fruits and veggies. *Organic* means that it has been grown without the pesticides that can transfer chemicals into the skin of the fruit or vegetable (that is, you can't just wash it off). A 2003 study from Seattle, Washington, compared how much pesticide contamination was absorbed into the bodies of preschool children who had eaten conventionally grown produce versus those who had eaten organic produce. The study found that the "total [organophosphorus pesticide breakdown of products] was approximately six times higher for children with conventional diets than for children with organic diets."

It's crazy that regular vegetables grown in the normal way are now considered "organic," which can mean special, fringe, and more expensive. But pesticide-sprayed apples show up in the bins as simply "apples." The same thing is true of genetically modified produce like corn and tomatoes. And yet, the produce that was grown from the earth without altered fish genes injected into them are sequestered in the organic section.

As reported by the FDA in the November/December issue of *FDA Consumer Magazine,* "The Grocery Manufacturers of America estimates that between 70 and 75 percent of all processed foods . . . may contain ingredients from genetically engineered plants." Are you shocked by those numbers? If so, that's because the food industry deliberately keeps that fact off food labels, because you wouldn't buy the product if they told you it was genetically modified. So it's hidden, and much money has been spent making sure it stays hidden. Given that, what do we do?

Remember that your health is not black or white—either or—but more like a continuous sliding scale. For example, let's say you grow all your own fruits and veggies, you have your own chickens in the yard, and your cattle out on the back forty are grass fed and slaughtered in the nicest possible way. All that would place you very high up on the health scale. If you washed down your chocolate-frosted cereal with soda for three meals every day, served with a side of fast food, you would be on the very low side of the scale.

Pick the best place on the scale you can, for your tastes and budget. If you're not ready to buy all organic produce and free-range meats, at least get the regular fruits and veggies and move yourself up on the health scale. If you can get organic or locally grown produce, do it. It's much better for you and you won't have to worry about just how much of the "pesticide breakdown products" are being absorbed by you or your children. But at the very least, don't buy faux foods. Find the place as high up on the scale as you personally can go. For example, in the case of fruit:

BEST: Organic fruit, locally grown.

ACCEPTABLE: Conventionally grown or genetically modified.

FAUX: Fruit-flavored products.

HOW OFTEN TO BUY: Purchase seasonal produce each time.

B. Prepared Foods

Typically, beside the deli and produce are the prepared foods. Many grocers now produce them: chicken cordon bleu, stuffed salmon, rotisserie chicken, sushi, and all kinds of healthy side dishes. They're wonderful if you're in a hurry. Just take them home, toss them into the oven, and, voilà, you're in business. The sides are good as well and, although it depends on the store, you can generally assume that the cole slaw is made with normal cabbage and mayonnaise, the hummus is real, and the macaroni salad is made from normal pasta. A store's products are more reliable because they don't need to use the food industry's chemicals. Their products don't have to withstand weeks of manufacture, packaging, and transportation only to last another two full weeks on the shelf.

This makes their prepared foods a perfect quick pickup for an easy dinner when your pantry's stock is low or you're out of time.

The only real drawback to these prepared foods concerns the meats used. It's impossible to know whether the salmon is farm raised, the tuna is mercury free, or the chicken is free range.

BEST: Veggie sides like hummus, cole slaw, and macaroni salad.

ACCEPTABLE: Main dishes such as sushi, prepared salmon, tuna, and chicken salads.

FAUX: Nothing here.

HOW OFTEN TO BUY: Whenever you are pressed for time and need something healthy, right away.

C. Deli

Deli meats are perfect for lunch sandwiches. In fact, most of the products you'll find in the deli case are just fine, but should be limited in quantity, from most frequently used to least frequently used in this order: turkey and chicken, ham, bologna, pepperoni, roast beef.

Again, real food is never the enemy, overconsumption of the food is what makes it bad. So the question is, for deli meats, where is the line? If you made ten trips to the deli, you might choose turkey or chicken five times, ham twice, and bologna, pepperoni, and roast beef once each.

The concern here is not the food itself, but the preservatives in it. However, many brands now produce nitrate-free varieties of their turkey, ham, and roast beef. Ask at the counter for them. If you shop at one of the grocery stores that feature natural and organic foods, such as Whole Foods, Wild Oats, and Trader Joe's, you'll have a better chance of finding them.

When choosing deli cheeses for your sandwich, avoid the items most likely to be hydrogenated—such as yellow and orange American singles. You can count on most Italian cheeses, including provolone and mozzarella. If in doubt, ask the person behind the counter to check the ingredients for you. Swiss is a variety that can go either way, so be sure to ask the attendant.

BEST: Any of the meats or cheeses, as long as they are nitrate-free and not made from hydrogenated oils.

ACCEPTABLE: Conventional deli meats, as long as you limit your consumption to once per week or less.

FAUX: Cheeses with hydrogenated oils.

HOW OFTEN TO BUY: Preservative-free deli meats and fresh cheeses are terrific staples to have on hand for emergency lunches, but the nitrate-laden varieties should be limited to once per week, and the hy-drogenated cheeses should never be substituted for the real thing.

D. Specialty Cheeses

What tradition could be more French than ending a meal with a fabu-lous cheese? But when you're shopping at a conventional store, many people have complained that they can't get anything better than the shrink-wrapped "mozzarella" sticks, "Parmesan" dust in a can, and "cheese food." But there's been something of a cheese awakening of late, and entirely new flavors are becoming more widely available in supermarkets across the country, from Brie and Camembert to goat cheeses, fetas, and even raw-milk varieties.

In fact, even some standard grocery stores now have so many choices that it seems overwhelming when you survey the mini-stadium of cheeses they line up for you. But have patience (this is the good part). Try new ones—or ask the attendant behind the counter to sneak you a little nibble so you can compare. Remember to buy smaller amounts than you think you need.

A little is wonderful. To keep from becoming unhealthy for you, simply don't eat a ton of it at once.

BEST: Almost all specialty cheeses are fine. But raw-milk cheeses will provide natural bacteria that are good for your digestive system.

ACCEPTABLE: The most mass-produced varieties will be more likely to use trace levels of artificial ingredients in their products. These are okay, but not as good as the cheeses made on smaller farms with all natural ingredients.

FAUX: None here. The fake cheeses are not sold in the specialty cheese area, they're over in the dairy section.

HOW OFTEN TO BUY: Make sure to buy small—because these calorie-dense nuggets should be eaten small as well, they will last a long time. If you buy in the smallest increment available, you could try a delicious new kind each week.

E. Fresh Breads

You are truly blessed and have been good in all your previous lives if your grocery store bakes fresh bread on-site—not the loaves wrapped in plastic. I'm talking about the ones that have been warm in recent memory and will go bad by the next day: your daily bread. (If you don't have access to fresh daily bread, see the recipe for Baguettes, page 298.)

Practice this habit when you're buying your bread: Pick up less than you think you'll need, so that you'll run out. If you have to throw away part of it because you didn't eat it all, buy a smaller loaf or baguette next time. This will help keep your consumption under control at home, and helps you to get in the habit of picking up fresh bread once or twice per week.

Any variety of fresh baked bread is enough to brighten your day, but you'll find yourself satisfied with smaller portions if you get the richer breads made with whole grains. Again, for recovering low-carb dieters, you don't *have* to eat whole-grain bread—there are no magic foods. But this variety will help keep you from being hungry two hours after eating.

Fresh bagels are fantastic, but please skip the doughnuts (bagels are cooked in water, doughnuts are cooked in a deep-fat fryer often filled with hydrogenated oils).

BEST: Fresh breads and bagels made on-site.

ACCEPTABLE: Fresh sweetened bread products such as coffee cakes and banana breads.

FAUX: Boxed coffee cakes, doughnuts, pastries, and pies.

HOW OFTEN TO BUY: You should have a little bread almost every day. If you indulge in coffee cake, doughnuts, or other sweetened products, do so only once per week at most.

F. Fish

Fish provide some of the best sources of healthy oils you can find, and taste great with white wine! So as you lay out your menu plan for the week, lean on fish. That said, faux foods lurk here, too. "Farm-raised fish" sounds wholesome—like apple pie, rosy cheeks, and straight white teeth. And the number of farm-raised fish and shellfish now account for about 15 percent of the total market. In fact, an incredible 70 million pounds of trout are grown on fish farms in the United States.

The process of growing farm-raised fish came under scrutiny when toxic chemicals were detected in them. Unfortunately, the issue of quality and contaminants and poisons in our food supply varies dramatically depending on who you talk to. The companies and industries making money selling farm-raised fish point to studies that say they are perfectly safe. Other studies say just the opposite. A July 2003 report from the Environmental Working Group pointed out that farm-raised salmon can harbor up to sixteen times more of the polychlorinated biphenyls (PCBs) than wild salmon (if you're still working through the faux-food concept, PCBs are definitely not a food).

But here's the irony. One reason the fish retain these harmful chemicals is precisely because of their wonderful healthy oils. That's where the PCBs happen to concentrate.

And then there's the dye that's injected into salmon flesh to make the salmon look as if they never needed to be injected with dye. Normal salmon eat shrimp and krill, and that turns their meat to a rosy coral color. Farm-raised fish are fed ground-up salmon, which leaves their flesh gray. So some marketing guru advised that the fish be injected with the chemicals canthaxanthin and astaxanthin to turn the salmon pink again. Magic. Canthaxanthin, in high quantities, has been associated with retinal damage in the human eye. The salmon industry says its fish, and the revenue stream they came from, are both safe.

What to do? Get wild-caught fish when you can. If you can't, remember that the concentration of contaminants in your body will depend on the volume you consume. Enjoy your fish, and eat small. By the way, the cheapest source for fresh-caught salmon is the stuff you find in the can.

BEST: Wild-caught or line-caught fish of any variety.

ACCEPTABLE: North American farm-raised fish is currently better than North Atlantic. Pressed imitation crabmeat is largely just leftover fish parts of unknown origin.

FAUX: Fish sticks and nuggets.

HOW OFTEN TO BUY: If you eat meat, fish should be one of your staples. A proper serving might be about one-third of a pound per person, and you should have some variety at least one or two times per week.

G. Pork

In the pork section, look for the leanest cuts. Pork chops make for wonderful, simple meals. They can be easily spiced and baked or sautéed in no time, and go perfectly with black beans, corn bread, any potatoes, broccoli . . . these are very versatile. A touch of pork sausage is lovely as a flavor enhancer for your spaghetti sauces, chilis, and gumbos. And most of the time these can be found as "Spicy" Italian or Cajun. If you love a little heat, you'll like these. Pork sausages should be enjoyed sparingly—certainly not every day.

BEST: Lean center-cut pork chops, tenderloin.

ACCEPTABLE: Pork sausage in moderation.

FAUX: Nothing faux here.

HOW OFTEN TO BUY: Keep enough on hand to have pork a couple of times per week. The sausage used for flavoring freezes very well, so just keep some on hand in your freezer. You will end up buying this once every few weeks.

H. Beef

A few years ago, the beef industry sued Oprah Winfrey because she doesn't really eat beef, and said so. Can you imagine? I'm glad they sued her. Who is she to not pander to a food industry? Who is she to have personal opinions of her own?

THE TRADITIONAL HEALTHY
MEDITERRANEAN DIET PYRAMID

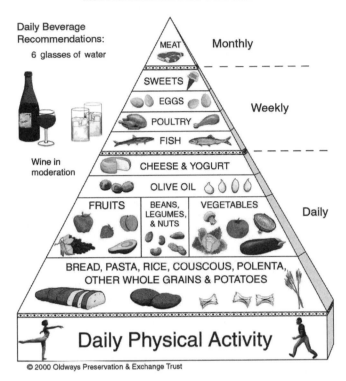

© 2000 Oldways Preservation & Exchange Trust

Perhaps the beef industry should start suing whole cultures as well. Mediterranean countries eat less beef than any other kind of meat. These are the thin, healthy people who outlive us and have fewer heart attacks. Can you imagine? Who are they to eat beef only once per month, maybe? Who are they to be so blatantly healthy, implying a link between healthy hearts and low beef consumption? Sue them all, I say.

According to the Mediterranean Diet Pyramid, put together by Oldways, the food issues think tank, and the Harvard School of Medicine, if you were to eat like these thin healthy people, you would avoid beef and have it only once every other week—if that! But don't tell anyone or the Texas lawyers will swagger up to your door, lawsuit in hand, for you and your healthy friends.

Moreover, the majority of U.S. cattle are typically given hormones to beef them up. These hormones include estradiol, progesterone, testosterone, zeranol, trenbolone acetate, and melengestiol acetate. The possibility that those hormones are retained within the meat should give anyone pause before picking it up. When you choose beef, avoid that with these bonus chemicals in them and get organic beef whenever you can.

BEST: Hormone-free beef, any cut.

ACCEPTABLE: Other varieties, conventionally raised, are not faux, but are not nearly as good for you as normal beef.

FAUX: Beef jerky.

HOW OFTEN TO BUY: Treat your beef like the French treat their entire approach to food—high quality, low quantity. Your beef should be very good, but eaten as an exception to your normal routine.

I. Chicken

The chicken section of the meat department has pieces, parts, and whole birds. Some of these will be "free range" and others will boast "no artificial ingredients." If the packages don't say anything at all, unfortunately, you can pretty much count on the fact that the birds were raised in a cage the size of your fist, force-fed, and injected with enough steroids to create the super chicken you see before you. It's not pretty, but it seems to have become the norm.

Like fish, you should rely on chicken as a staple meat—just try to avoid the injected birds. Most people live their lives struggling to cope with the hormones they have on board naturally. Don't add to your worries. You don't need those chemicals in your chicken, and then in your body, and especially not in your children.

BEST: Free-range chickens and those produced without artificial ingredients.

ACCEPTABLE: Birds with no artificial ingredients.

FAUX: If it doesn't say free-range . . . and it doesn't say "no artificial ingredients" . . . you should avoid it.

HOW OFTEN TO BUY: Chicken should be one of your principle meats, and you should have it as often as one or two times per week.

J. Nitrate Depot: Preserved Pork

Laminated sausage products will be the food of choice for a nuclear winter. In fact, this whole section of kielbasa-like products *can* be eaten healthily, but must be done so very sparingly. The nitrates used as preservatives have been associated with a number of health problems, and are completely unnecessary (see Appendix II: A Rogue's Gallery of Faux-Food Additives).

How much can you have? Two bacon slices at breakfast is plenty, no more. And you shouldn't have bacon with your breakfast more than twice per week. The Scottish and Irish have some of the highest heart disease rates in this region of the galaxy, and tend to eat bacon every day. You do the math.

BEST: If you can find nitrate-free bacon (and this is actually available now), this would be your best bet. Freshly made sausage from your butcher or, in some cases, from right there in your grocery store meat section, is wonderful because it does not have to be spiked with preservatives.

ACCEPTABLE: All standard bologna, hot dog, and sausage products in this section are acceptable, if barely.

FAUX: Prepackaged lunch packets with processed meat, hydrogenated-oil crackers, and faux cheese spread should be avoided altogether.

HOW OFTEN TO BUY: Shrink-wrapped pork products should be purchased no more than once every other week, but you should shoot for buying them only monthly at best.

K. Dairy Products

Milk, sour cream, buttermilk, cream, and half-and-half are all healthy choices that have the added benefit of being delicious. Try buttermilk when you bake (see the recipe for Somebody's Buttermilk Biscuits, page 300), half-and-half in your coffee, and sour cream in your mashed potatoes or chili. Milk's calcium, as we know, is terrific for the health of your teeth, bones, and even for weight loss.

If you like low-fat milk products, or have concerns about normal milk, keep in mind that there's nothing inherently wrong with drinking the low-fat variety. But it tastes thin, so typically you'll need to consume more of it to satisfy you—good for the food industry, bad for you. Normal milk will satisfy you more with less volume, and helps you make the transition to the low quantity–high quality approach to eating.

If you don't want to drink organic milk, whatever you do, don't try this experiment. Don't have someone fill two identical glasses, one with organic milk and the other with milk from regular mass-produced, hormone-injected cows—and then do a blind taste test between them. What you won't be noticing when you don't do this experiment is the overwhelming difference between them. Hormone milk tastes watery (as if they're forcing more out of the cow than it was made to give). Organic milk tastes full and delicious. And once you know this, you can't "unknow" it, and it's very hard to go back to the flavorless milk.

The hormone injected into cows to make them produce more milk is genetically engineered recombinant bovine growth hormone (rBGH). That milk can be laced with hormones (insulin-like growth factor 1, or IGF-1) that you certainly don't need. Don't bother reading the label for a warning either—the people who make it don't want you to know that you're drinking milk from their chemo-cows. Again, here's where the sliding scale comes in again. It's better for you than soda, but not nearly as good as organic.

BEST: Organic dairy products.

ACCEPTABLE: Conventional dairy products, with the proviso that normal levels of milk fat will satisfy you more on less volume than the low-fat versions.

FAUX: Any dairy product such as low-fat half-and-half or nondairy creamer spiked with high-fructose corn syrup is definitely faux.

HOW OFTEN TO BUY: The French, as adults, don't actually drink milk. So if you were to be rigorous about living their lifestyle, you would never have it, and get your calcium from cheese and yogurt. But I see nothing unhealthy about moderate consumption. Organic milk, in my house, is kept in stock at all times.

L. Eggs

Here's a complete fallacy that we've believed forever. Ready? The cholesterol you eat shuttles straight into your blood, clogs your arteries, and increases your risk of dropping dead from a heart attack. This notion, it turns out, is a myth.

Need more information? Dr. Walter Willett, analyzing data from the Nurses' Health Study II, has shown that you can eat one to two eggs per day (diabetics aside), without raising your likelihood of having a heart attack. Even better, the changes you do see in blood cholesterol actually indicate that eggs improve your ratio of "good" HDL to "bad" LDL cholesterol. The higher your HDL cholesterol—and the lower your LDL cholesterol—the better.

Here's the take-home message: You don't have to be afraid of eggs anymore. They're the most nutrient dense of all foods with an absolute trove of health benefits. The French eat eggs nearly every day, don't have our heart problems, and these healthy people are certainly not eating "egg products," egg substitutes, egg remainders or any other silliness. In fact, no one else on the planet is eating fake eggs except us, the overweight, unhealthy people.

Have you ever compared organic eggs to "regular"? The yolks of the organic eggs tend to sit higher in the whites, which tend to be clearer. Of course, everything depends on the particular factory your grocers get their eggs from, but in general, organic eggs will be better.

BEST: Eggs, organically grown.

ACCEPTABLE: Conventional eggs.

FAUX: Egg substitute has an incredible 444 milligrams of sodium per serving. That's almost 20 percent of your recommended daily allowance for the entire day, in one serving.

HOW OFTEN TO BUY: Normal eggs should be in your refrigerator at all times—not just for eating, but also for sauces and baking as well.

M. Butter

Margarine has been around since the 1800s and was invented, ironically, by the French. Today, of course, they won't touch it (I think they just wanted to sell it to the rest of us). The benefit of margarine for industrial food products is that it makes them more nonbiodegradable. *Bacteria* won't even eat it—think about this. The shelf life of hydrogenated oil in your kitchen is listed as "indefinite" with no need to refrigerate it. The shelf life of motor oil is indefinite, with no need to refrigerate it. The shelf life of plastic . . . you get the picture.

By contrast, butter has nutrients like vitamin A, vitamin E, and selenium, all of which are vastly better for your heart than anything found in margarine. The concern with butter is that it contains saturated fats, but the Harvard School of Public Health has recently announced that hydrogenated oils (most commonly found in margarine and Crisco) are even more dangerous for your heart than saturated fats. And the hydrogenated oils do not have the benefits of the heart-healthy vitamins and minerals found quite naturally in plain butter.

And in countries like France, where they eat saturated fats every single day in the form of butters and cheeses and yogurts and creams, they still have fewer heart attacks than us. A principle difference in their butter consumption is that their food volume is quite small. So the rule is the same for butter as it is for every other fabulous food. If you eat a vat of it, it can be unhealthy. If you have a little, you get the health *benefits*. In this line of thinking, butter is not a problem unless you and I make it one with our eating patterns. We'll go over this in detail in Steps 5 to 7, when we learn the *how* of eating.

One last thing: Buy unsalted butter. I learned this at a "convivium" of the Slow Food Society, in which we had an extensive butter-tasting afternoon, with expert chefs and representatives from local dairies. I was surprised to learn that salt is added to butter simply as a preservative to keep inferior batches of cream from going from marginal to worse. The better cream doesn't need the salt, so remains unsalted.

BEST: Real butter, unsalted.

ACCEPTABLE: Salted butter.

FAUX: Margarine or any other butter substitute.

HOW OFTEN TO BUY: Butter should be a staple that you have on hand for cooking and baking at all times.

N. Fake Breads

You've seen them. The rows of shiny plastic-wrapped sliced breads, and not one of them has fewer than ten ingredients. They can't just include normal ingredients because the loaves would go bad too soon, the company would lose money, go out of business, and then you'd have to get your bread fresh from a bakery.

In this row you find sliced breads, bagels, English muffins, pita, and everything in between. In general, if there are fresh, real food varieties of these products, they're not shelved in this section.

BEST: Fresh baked goods, which you'll not likely find here.

ACCEPTABLE: Some varieties may have no other faux ingredients, but you'll have to dig to identify them.

FAUX: The lot.

HOW OFTEN TO BUY: Never buy chemically preserved breads with hydrogenated oil.

O. Freezer Desserts

Of the millions of desserts, confections, and toppings in the store's freezers, only two are decent: quality ice cream and 100 percent fruit pops. The ice cream, however, should have only a handful of ingredients, such as plain Breyers. Though even this brand has many new products with an unpronounceable litany of fillers that seem at odds with their original mission to produce products with "ingredients that Johnny can read."

Fruit pops are fine if they're made with 100 percent fruit, but the slurry of corn syrup and hydrogenated oil you'll find in this aisle is ridiculous. You can make whipped cream at home in thirty-seven seconds—check out the recipe for Vanilla Whipped Cream (page 329). It's dirt simple, and you can flavor it any way you like. You can also make your own fruit pops at home with 100 percent fruit juice, and the taste is better than any faux-food concoction you can shake a Popsicle stick at.

BEST: Ice cream with fewer than six ingredients, all of which you can read and understand. Popsicles sweetened with 100 percent fruit juice.

ACCEPTABLE: Fruit pops sweetened with sugar or cane juice.

FAUX: Most ice cream bars, "healthy" ice creams, and whipped toppings.

HOW OFTEN TO BUY: Ice cream is a perfect dessert, when eaten in small amounts. Real ice cream should be a stock item in your freezer. Fruit pops are fantastic summer desserts for kids (and dads when no one's looking!).

P. Frozen Fruits and Vegetables

Frozen vegetables are great. They're no less healthy than the fresh ones, may be more cost effective, and they're convenient to boot. They won't taste as good as fresh, but many times you're putting these frozen veggies in something else anyway (like pot pie or casseroles).

Frozen french fries, however, usually taste like they're 5 percent real potatoes and 95 percent filler. Unless the ingredients stop at "potatoes," you have no idea what they've spritzed on their spuds.

French fries have gotten a nutritional black eye because food companies manipulate the texture of potatoes with chemicals called alginates, and "flavor enhancers" to mimic the desirable flavor of beef tallow. Even when these potato products reach the restaurant, they're cooked in partially hydrogenated oils.

It's easy to make your own french fries. Cut up a potato at home, throw it in a pan with some olive oil, and sauté it until it's just done. Made fresh, these become just another formerly forbidden health food you can enjoy any time you want. Baked or fried, spiced as you like, and they're a million times healthier. Plus they take only a few minutes to throw together (about the same amount of time it takes to heat up faux fries in the oven).

If you can find frozen dinners worth eating, you're probably an archeologist. If you must have a frozen dinner, read the label. Unless it says, "nothing artificial, and this prepackaged pot pie contains less sodium than Salt Lake City, Utah," don't buy it. You can do it better and tastier at home. The same is true for frozen pizza. (See the recipes for Healthful Pepperoni Pizza, page 294, and Chicken Potpie, page 283.)

Frozen fruits, like frozen veggies, are great in baked dishes. Blueberries, raspberries, and strawberries make great cobblers, fruit sauces, and additions to your morning yogurt.

BEST: Frozen fruit, such as blueberries and raspberries. Frozen veggies, such as peas, corn, and beans.

ACCEPTABLE: I have seen some frozen dinners that are not loaded with faux-food ingredients, and they taste okay. You'll just have to look hard for them.

FAUX: Most frozen dinners, pot pies, potato products, and pizzas.

HOW OFTEN TO BUY: Frozen fruits are a stock item for your morning yogurts, for fruit sauces, and even for fruit cobblers (see the recipe for Cuppa Cuppa Cuppa Apple Cobbler, page 319). Purchase your frozen veggies only as you need them for an upcoming dish.

Q. Cereals

Have you ever been in a carnival exhibit where mirrors were placed at opposite sides of a room? When you enter, you appear to be replicated on and on into infinity. This is what it looks like when you turn into "cereal row" and have to choose something from the grinning painted clowns, green leprechauns, chocolate vampires, and tigers in groovy bandanas.

As we know, all the candy, cookie, and frosted cereals are deliberately placed on the bottom row to better bait our children at eye-level. The aisle itself is placed roughly in the center of the store so that, by the time you get there, the child is tired enough to be primed for a good bout of whining.

Don't be fooled by the boxes of cookies, s'mores, and marshmallow rice cereals that claim something like "part of a balanced breakfast because we threw a multivitamin in there." If you absolutely have to get cereal for you kids, ordinary Cheerios are not too bad because they contain whole grain oats, plain sugar (fourth ingredient), and a multivitamin. Alternatively, you could pick up some regular oats and make oatmeal (see the recipe for Brown Sugar Cinnamon Oatmeal, page 272). The little powdered packets of oats are normally filled with disturbing ingredients. Regular oats are fine. Plain granola (Kashi makes a good one) makes a great breakfast with fruit and yogurt.

BEST: Grains such as oats, grits, and wheat cereals. These are fantastic and can be prepared in the way you like best.

ACCEPTABLE: Boxed cereals with no hydrogenated oils, high-fructose corn syrup, or dyes, such as regular Cheerios.

FAUX: Instant packets of oats, most cereals.

HOW OFTEN TO BUY: Cereals are a staple to keep in your cupboard for a quick and easy breakfast.

R. Condiments

In the next step, we'll be talking about easy ways to lose weight by losing your sweet tooth. One of the easiest ways to curb your sugar craving is this: Give up store-bought ketchup. Its high-fructose corn syrup feeds your sweet tooth and activates cravings for other overtly sweetened foods (although a few ketchup brands are now made with natural sweeteners). Mustards are wonderful and make fantastic additions to sauces and vinaigrette dressings (we've included a few super simple recipes that take all of five minutes to throw together). Mayonnaise, if made with eggs, vegetable oil, spices, and lemons, is wonderful (see the recipe for A Mayonnaise of Your Very Own, page 259).

Make sure your jellies or jams are 100 percent fruit, and that your peanut butter has no partially hydrogenated oil or zinc oxide in it. Smuckers makes a good one that contains only peanuts and salt. Even better, you can find stores where they grind the peanuts on site.

BEST: Any mustard, 100 percent real fruit jams, peanut butter with no more than two ingredients, any Tabasco or plain horseradish, olive spreads, hummus, and regular mayonnaise.

ACCEPTABLE: Horseradish "sauces," canola mayonnaise.

FAUX: Reduced-fat mayonnaise, peanut butter with hydrogenated oil, and jams with corn syrup.

HOW OFTEN TO BUY: These should be staples in your cupboard and refrigerator.

S. Baking Aisle

Please don't buy the can of hydrogenated oil called shortening. Why bake with something that contributes to heart disease?

As for white flour and white sugar, we have to talk about our obsession with "white." What is it with this color? Food manufacturers strip all the healthy parts of the grain from their flour, just so it can look white. And they even bleach it, as if removing the nutrients were a good thing. Sugar refineries strip the minerals from the sugar so it can look . . . white. They even sell something called "brownulated" sugar, which is just brown sugar with extra caramel color added. Unbelievable.

Although there's nothing particularly unhealthy about white flour, when the whole grains are stripped out, there aren't many vitamins and minerals left. The same is true for white sugar. So when you choose your flour or sugar, be sure to choose the darker varieties whenever possible. For example, have you ever looked at the back of a molasses jar? It's a fantastic health food. A single tablespoon has 20 percent of all the calcium you need for an entire day, 20 percent of the iron, and 20 percent of the potassium (a potassium-rich diet has been shown to help reduce hypertension).

Bittersweet chocolate should always have a revered place in your cupboard, at least for Hot Cocoa (page 270) and chocolate truffles. It's a wonderful health food and you need to have just a little every day. Make it dark chocolate and eat it as an ender, described in Step 4. If you do that, you'll get the heart-healthy polyphenols of the cocoa. Don't get cheap chocolate or chocolate bars with the nougat, wafers, and other fillers in them. Make chocolate your favorite health food by just eating the chocolate. Keep the amount you eat at any one time down to about two thumbs (see Step 4).

Another staple of this section is extra-virgin olive oil. When you need a lighter oil for pancakes or muffins or something like that, use 100 percent vegetable oil.

BEST: Extra-virgin olive oil, whole-wheat flour, molasses, dark brown sugar, bittersweet chocolate, cocoa.

ACCEPTABLE: White sugar, white flour, semisweet chocolate.

FAUX: Bisquick, cocoa mix, "brownulated" sugar.

HOW OFTEN TO BUY: Flour should be in your cupboard all the time, as should baking chocolate, cocoa, olive oil, and brown sugar.

T. Canned Fruits and Vegetables

Look for the canned vegetables that do not contain added sugars. For example, in my local grocery store, only one brand of canned corn (out of four) was free of syrup. Why in the world would you put syrup in corn? We like to buy spiced beans for our chili, but had to sort through the brands before we found the one with the least ingredients and no added sugar at all. That's the one you want. In addition, canned veggies are also more likely to have added salt.

Most of the canned vegetables you'll use on a daily basis will be beans (white, black, pinto, and field peas), which can be spiced up and ready to eat in no time. Canned tomatoes, tomato sauce, and tomato paste are easily used as a base for chili, spaghetti sauce, and tomato-based soups. As for the others, canned mushrooms taste like *sole de la shoe* compared to fresh, and canned green beans and asparagus are so dishwater insipid that it's no wonder an entire generation has grown up hating vegetables. So get these fresh and sauté them in a pan. It's a breeze, and they'll taste terrific.

BEST: Any canned beans or tomatoes with no more than two ingredients (tomatoes and salt, for example), fruit packed in water, or 100 percent fruit juice.

ACCEPTABLE: Canned veggies like mushrooms and asparagus often taste horrible, but are not explicitly bad for you and might go well in some dishes, such as Hot Artichoke-Cheese Dip (page 257).

FAUX: Any with corn syrup, or more than 5 percent of your daily requirement of sodium per serving.

HOW OFTEN TO BUY: Canned beans and tomatoes should be in your cupboard all the time, for recipes such as The Last Lasagna (page 278), but you don't need to have canned fruit unless you're making a particular dish that calls for it.

U. Alcohol

State laws are quirky regarding alcohol in grocery stores. Some won't let anything but cough syrup and vanilla flavoring through their doors. Some allow beer and others sell wine and even spirits, so you don't have to make multiple trips. When your shopping involves beer or wine, there are a few things to keep in mind.

Before I tell you that alcohol does what aspirin does (prevents platelet accumulation), and that beer and wine provide health benefits (great B vitamins, great for your heart, great antioxidants), I have to be conservative and say that some people can have trouble keeping their quantity small. Just as with butter, eggs, sugars, and everything else, a little may be good for you, but a lot is not. This is especially true with alcohol. If you don't think you can hold your consumption to just one to two drinks per day, don't even start. Switch to grape juice or cocoa to get your polyphenols.

Disclaimer done, now on to the health information.

Dark beer has been shown to reduce homocystene, a factor associated with heart disease. Guinness, for example, is great for you—sort of like liquid bread. Wine is like vitamin W, famously packed with antioxidants and flavonols that protect your heart. Red is better than white, not only because of its nutritional properties, but also because you tend to sip red wine rather than gulp it, and this helps you practice the habits of eating and drinking small. Other alcohols are okay, but the best benefits come from dark beer and red wine.

BEST: Dark beer, red wine.

ACCEPTABLE: Light beer, white and sweet wines.

FAUX: Oversweetened wine coolers.

HOW OFTEN TO BUY: If you have a little wine or beer with your dinner, you should buy according to your proclivities. If you only cook with wine or sherry, you will purchase these once a month or so.

V. Coffee and Tea

In the 1950s, researchers suggested a link between caffeine and cancer, which has been repeated in the media many times. But this study was found to be flawed, and this link has since turned out to be completely false. In fact, in the massive Nurses' Health Study II, Harvard's Walter Willett investigated whether cancer is related to caffeine consumption. He found that "during almost 2 million person-years of follow-up, 1,438 cases of colorectal cancer were observed. Consumption of caffeinated coffee or tea intake was not associated with the incidence of colon or rectal cancer." In addition, other research has found that coffee or tea drinkers were far less likely to have indications of liver disfunction than people who abstained.

So it's time to move on. Sure, get the decaf if regular coffee makes you jittery, but know that regular coffee is perfectly fine. But please note: To emulate the healthy French habits, you're allowed coffee that comes only in a normal-size cup, not the the venti mambo Big Gulp. Always buy the small size. Tea is equally wonderful, is loaded with heart-healthy polyphenols, and you're free to choose the kind you enjoy most.

BEST: Regular coffee and tea that comes in bags or loose.

ACCEPTABLE: Decaffeinated coffee, flavored herbal teas.

FAUX: Instant flavored coffee mixes and bottled "tea drinks" with high-fructose corn syrup.

HOW OFTEN TO BUY: To your tastes. Keep in mind that you do not have to drink coffee just because the French do, or tea for that matter. When you have it by the small cup, you'll end up purchasing this product sparingly.

W. Boxed Foods

Some boxed foods are fine, like plain pasta and natural rice pilaf. But the mac and cheese with the Yellow No. 6 packet of powder should be replaced by making it at home. Whipping together a delicious macaroni and cheese is so easy, can be done on the stove, and takes no longer than the typical cardboard variety (see the recipe on page 307).

Most of the "helper" foods are best left on the shelf with the instant au gratin potatoes. Again, these taste much better when made at home, and aren't hard to throw together. Just check the ingredients on the back of the box if you have questions about whether something is a food or not.

BEST: Plain pasta, rice, 100 percent natural pilafs, and risottos.

ACCEPTABLE: Boxed grains (pilaf, couscous, and so on) with spice packets.

FAUX: Most "helper" boxed products, any of the boxed potato products, Rice-A-Roni–type foods, and any rice and sauce packets.

HOW OFTEN TO BUY: Keep natural pilafs and risottos on hand. They're great for a quick addition to the meal. Pasta is also a must to stock in the cupboard for those nights when you have no idea what you're going to have (see the recipe for pizza sauce, page 295).

X. Soda and Drinks

Unless you're picking up seltzer water, which you can mix with 100 percent juice if you want a bubbly drink, don't even visit this aisle. Diet drinks are just as bad, because of the chemical sweeteners like aspartame and phosphoric acid. You must cut these out altogether. If you do nothing other than give up these drinks, you'll take weight off and improve your health. If you want something in a bottle around the house, have water.

Be careful when choosing juice. Some labels blare FRUIT JUICE in seventy-two-point, extra-bold type, but the juice is really only 10 percent of the total. This means they are 90 percent dyed syrup with some cranberries waved over the top of the vat before being trucked to the bottling plant. If you want juice, get juice. If you want syrup, get syrup. Just don't confuse the two!

Sport drinks: You're told that your physiology constantly teeters on the edge of a disastrous electrolyte imbalance and, with any exertion at all, you're going to need immediate replenishment. This may be true if you've just swum the English Channel, finished an Ironman competition, or been stranded in Death Valley for a day. Even at that, it makes no sense at all to replace them with a neon vehicle for high-fructose corn syrup.

Sweetened teas and flavored waters are additional confusions to watch out for in this aisle. You don't need to drink your calories, and you don't need to feed your sweet tooth with these drinks either. Stick with regular tea and regular water.

BEST: Water, 100 percent fruit drinks.

ACCEPTABLE: Naturally sweetened teas.

FAUX: Any drink with high-fructose corn syrup and dye in it—which means just about all of them, in bottles or sold as powders.

HOW OFTEN TO BUY: Bottled water and juice are good to keep around, especially if you have concerns about what's coming out of your tap. As for the other choices, unless you're Lance Armstrong and have just pedaled over the Pyrenees, you don't need them, ever.

Y. Chips and Snacks

Since the increased awareness that hydrogenated oils contribute to heart disease, food manufacturers have been looking for alternatives. This is the power of people voting with their shopping carts. The way to continue this trend in the snacks section is to buy chips with nonhydrogenated oils or those that are baked. Unfortunately, we're still hard-pressed to find pretzels or crackers without these heart-harming oils.

Plain popcorn—not popcorn from a bag—is a great snack because the ingredients read: corn kernels. You just put them in a pot with a couple tablespoons of vegetable oil, throw a lid on, and shake until all the kernels are popped. It's easy, there are no chemicals for your body to fight off, and it's great entertainment for kids. Unsalted nuts are also fantastic snacks. The extra salt is unnecessary, can contribute to hypertension, and also makes you crave more later.

If they're not in the snacks section, look for dried fruits by the produce. They make wonderful nibbles or additions to your morning yogurt: raisins, dried plums, apricots, figs, cranberries, cherries, and bananas. Throw these in a bag with some brazil nuts or cashews and you've got a righteous trail mix.

BEST: Plain popcorn, unsalted nuts, baked chips, dried fruits.

ACCEPTABLE: Salted nuts, lightly sugared berries such as cranberries.

FAUX: Bagged popcorn, flavored potato chips, and chips with hydrogenated oils.

HOW OFTEN TO BUY: Snacks should be a rarity. Purchase perhaps once every other week.

Z. Checkout

Is there ever anything of redeeming value in the impulse aisle? Think about it for just a minute. "Bat-Boy Emerges from Hell to Terrorize Small Texas Hamlet." "Are Jen and (fill in the blank) on the Verge of Divorce?" Thirty-two colors of Tic Tacs crowd the Life Savers and sorbitol gum. It's a circus in that space, from one end to the other.

I know it's fun to buy things, especially when you're bored and waiting for the woman in front of you to figure out how to work the auto teller. But you'll get more nutritional value by eating the "Bat-Boy Emerges from Hell" article than you will from anything in the impulse aisle.

BEST: If you're lucky, you might be able to find a quality dark chocolate here, but most of these items are less healthful than the Duracell batteries they're next to.

ACCEPTABLE: Nothing, really.

FAUX: Chewing gum tape, candies, mouth cracklin' poppers, the zoo of gummy animals. All of it.

HOW OFTEN TO BUY: You don't need these, and neither do your children.

Troubleshooting

Expect that your first two trips to the store will take some reorientation. You have to change how you read labels as you learn to avoid faux foods and bring home real foods. But by the third trip out, you'll have already found the few cereals of any nutritional value, and you'll have identified the healthy cheeses and the canned vegetables without corn syrup in them. At that point, it's a piece of cake!

Don't be swayed by the advertisements for the products you always thought were healthful, like those low-fat foods with synthetic sugars and oils, or the "real fruit juice" imposters, or the "fresh" breads wrapped in plastic with thirty-two ingredients in them. Make sure the foods you bring home are real foods.

It's best to go shopping by yourself at first, so you can keep to your resolve. If you go with your children (or spouse), you might be tempted to buy Pop-Tarts because of the picture of a blueberry on the box. Remember, if you don't bring home faux foods, they won't get eaten.

Don't Forget, Don't Diet

When you bring home your grocery bags full of real food for the first time, expect your dieting instincts to rear their ugly heads. *I've got so many carbs here,* you'll fret. You'll momentarily consider the foods you've purchased to evaluate which has the lowest amount of fat. But recognize these thoughts for what they are, and push them out of your mind. You have permission not to diet, and to eat wonderful foods again. And once you realize how easy it is to shop for real foods and taste how delicious they are, you honestly won't miss the dieting approach of scrutinizing the RDA microfiche on the back of the little boxes.

Remember, too, that this entire luscious lifestyle approach exchanges high quantity for high-quality foods. So when you shop, buy the best you can find, just get less of it. You'll be just as satisfied, you'll have better nutrition, and you'll lose weight in the process.

I want you to notice how your physiology responds to this French approach—not only with increased energy levels and lower weight, but also in the kinds of foods your body begins to crave. A wonderful benefit of eating real food again is that you begin to lose your need for oversweetened junk foods. Your tastes acclimate to the higher quality.

In fact, the next step on this path shows you how your transformation of tastes occurs, and how this one change creates a lifetime of optimal health.

❦ People on The PATH

Dear Will,

I just want to say that your book has changed my life! I have gone from a size 24/26 to a 6. That's right—a size SIX. I am just under 5'4" and used to weigh 235 pounds. Right now, I weigh 130 pounds.

I have struggled with my weight all my life and feel as if I've found the ultimate answer to my struggles. I basically began incorporating changes that fit well with my family life, my budget, and my personal preferences. For instance, you will never catch me drinking soda (I think I'd throw up!) or eating a low-fat food product (normal fat all the way for me).

By the way, I am a thirty-one-year-old, stay-at-home mother of four children and my weight loss is the talk of the town. People I run into who haven't seen me in a while hardly recognize me. I began eating this way in August 2003 and I plan to do this for the rest of my life. I'm sure you've heard this before, but THANK YOU for creating your eating plan. I think it probably saved my life.

All of the changes I made are from following your advice.

Thanks again,

Joy H

CHEAT SHEET: Fabulous Foods

Make a fresh beginning. This new introduction of real foods is the biological jump start your body has been asking for. Go to the store and refill your cabinets with the healthy choices that give you the best possible nutrition and the best possible shot at lifelong health.

You still have to read labels, but not for fats, carbs, and proteins. Instead, you'll be looking for real foods with real ingredients. Get used to shopping for:

- Organic veggies
- Organic meats

- Normal dairy products
- Packaged foods that are 100 percent natural

The Results You're Looking For

IMMEDIATELY

- You'll notice the dramatic improvement in the flavor of your foods.
- You will look forward to dinner.

WITHIN TWO WEEKS

- You'll have mapped out the real foods in your grocery store and shopping will be a breeze.

WITHIN A MONTH

- The real foods you're choosing will seem perfectly normal, and the faux foods you used to eat will taste bizarre by comparison.

HOMEWORK: FINDING THE FAUX IN YOUR HOUSE

1. Map the grocery store.
   a. Learn which aisles have real foods in them.
   b. Learn which aisles do not.
2. Try organic meats and judge the difference for yourself.
3. Get organic veggies whenever you can.
4. Taste test the difference between organic milk and chemically treated milk.

Lose Your Sweet Tooth
(While Eating Real Chocolate)

At ten years old, my son Ben was already a discriminating individual with a very secure sense of WIIFM ("What's in it for me?"). So when we said we were going to live in France for a while (and he shrugged), I had to arm myself with the full parental arsenal of reasons why living in this other culture would be so cool.

What a failure. None of it worked: culture (whatever), a new language (major yawn), and the "exciting adventure" even sounded lame to me the moment it came out of my mouth. But what finally changed his little teen-wanna-be brain was food. Not just any food. Chocolate.

"Ben," I intoned, "you know, they eat chocolate croissants for breakfast." Now that got his attention. He squinted, digesting this little mental anomaly. Surely there must be some trick, some broccoli laced within, or some other suffering-induced builder of character.

"Chocolate? For breakfast?"

There it was. The opening. The French were potentially cool, so I used ever so little parental license and pushed the truth envelope. "Yeah, um, I think they have it every day!" I knew I had him when he finally started with the gentle bobble-headed movements he makes when he's on board with you. We had him.

Okay, the French don't have chocolate for breakfast every day, but you can pick up a *pain au chocolat* any morning you and your parents like! This particular fact really hits hard on another version of the French paradox (there are so many). "The French eat those croissants, those chocolates! How can they have all these sweet foods without their insulin levels (and weight) going through the roof?"

But if you've ever stopped at a local French bakery and picked up a croissant, you know that they're far less sugary than buttery. The chocolate is mostly darker and richer, without so much sugar, and the yogurts don't contain buckets of corn syrup either. By the way, there's no equivalent to the milk shake macchiato "coffee" drinks we have here.

In fact, the French can eat those wonderful breads, chocolates, and pastries precisely because they *aren't* spiked with so much sugar. It's not dumped in there because they just don't have the insatiable taste for it like you find in other (heavier) cultures. Isn't that a coincidence? They don't have our cultural sweet tooth or our cultural weight problems.

Our taste for more and more sugar in our foods is a basic craving that reflects how much you want. But that much sweetness in food spins your body out of control and into weight and health problems by producing disordered eating. In this step, you'll get the tools to regain control over your cravings again.

The first place to start is with sugar. We eat piles of it, particularly in processed food products. We're saturated with it. The USDA reported that Americans eat twice the maximum sugar they should be getting from their diets—about twenty teaspoons every day! Of course, much of this is hidden in all the fake food products out there—practically all fat-free and processed foods have some form of corn syrup in them.

Your goal to eat like the French: Cut sugar consumption by half by *changing your taste for it,* not by cutting sugar out of natural foods.

Here's where the loss of control comes in. People say they eat sugar because they crave it. In other words, because they have a sweet tooth. And that sweet tooth calls them and nags them for sugary treats. But this confuses cause with effect. The sweet tooth didn't create the consumption of sweets, the consumption of sweets created the tooth.

This point is easier to understand by thinking of an addict of any stripe. Addicts seek out their fix because they crave it, but they crave it in the first place because they used it. Your body naturally gets used to the inputs you give it—Ding Dongs and Jolly Ranchers all day long, let's say. It responds by expecting that threshold level of sweetness until you change the baseline.

Fortunately, losing your sweet tooth is easy to do, by removing the excess sugar in your life. I'm not talking about eliminating carbs or healthy fruits with natural sweetness, but those products with additive sugars. This one simple habit will tone down the sensitivity of your taste for sugar, so you just won't want so much anymore.

Right now, you have a sense of the sweetness that certain foods carry. Some, like a chicken breast, are not sweet at all. Some have a little sweetness, like bread (the enzymes in your mouth break down the complex carbs into simple carbs, and you taste a subtle sweetness). Then there's dark chocolate, fruits like bananas, milk chocolate, sweeter fruits like peaches, and on up to sodas and candy.

All the way from "not sweet at all" to "makes me gag," your personal assessment is related to the relative size of your sweet tooth. If it's large, you'll taste syrupy soda and think it tastes normal. If your tooth has been just about pulled out, you'll taste that very same soda and be overwhelmed by the sugar concentration. Your mission, should you choose to accept it, is to move your taste for sugars from point A to point B.

And here's the message of hope. Many people really believe they're controlled by their urges, and driven to bad eating habits by their tastes for certain foods. But you can set your sweetness sensitivity anywhere you want.

For example, when my daughter Grace was in third grade, I gave her elementary school teachers a series of PATH Healthy Weight Loss seminars from Thanksgiving to Valentine's Day, to show them that you really can lose weight, even through the eating frenzy of the holidays.

One of the teachers was a Pepsi-aholic, and drank 3 or 4 cans per day. For a hundred health reasons, she was finally convinced to kick the habit and give soda up for good. She stopped cold turkey.

Three weeks later, she came to the course with a personal revelation. "Dr. Clower, I was home the other day. My son was sitting at the computer with a bag of Hershey's kisses right right beside him—*open*. I went over to chat and absentmindedly stuck my hand in the bag and pulled out one as we talked. After I finished that piece of chocolate, I was 'sweeted out.' I didn't want any more! Three weeks ago, I would have had ten of those things without even blinking."

This woman lost her sweet tooth in three weeks by making one basic change that reduced her sugar consumption. Three weeks later, her tolerance for sweetness had dramatically dropped as her sensitivity to sugary tastes increased. And the most important fact is that she's now doing all the right things for all the right reasons.

Now she's making healthy food decisions based on what she loves.

Now she's controlling calories based on her taste and instincts.

Now she's living the French lifestyle that produces low weight for her, even when she's not thinking about it.

And just like the French people, she no longer has to agonize about her diet, calculate fat grams as a percentage of total calorie consumption, or stew over the number of hydrogens saturating the fatty acid chains of her mashed potatoes. And the best part is that she did this herself, and knows how to do it again if she ever needs to. She's empowered to control her own cravings so she can live a healthy, enjoyable life.

When you see the naturally thin French people eat pleasantly without overconsumption, realize that you really can do that, too. You can get there through your own behaviors and choices because you can change what your body craves. You're in control of this aspect of your life.

Remember, the point is not just about calories or carbs or even your weight! You're cutting the sugar to regain control over your cravings, so that your natural tendency is toward optimal health. Once you do this, you change your relationship with food, enjoy it more, and (as a wonderful consequence) you lose weight.

The Sweet Tooth Test

To lose your sweet tooth, you first have to get a sense of how intense it is right now. Once you have a measurement, you can watch your sugar craving changes over time. That's where the sweet tooth test comes in—it's a quick test and I advocate taking it once a week for the next two months.

The Test

What you need:

> 5 small cups, all of the same size
> Corn syrup (Karo or another kind) or sugar
> A notebook to track your results

1. Get your five small cups and fill each two-thirds full with water. The size of the cups doesn't matter. Just make sure they're the same cups you use every time you take this test. The first cup will be a reference cup, and contain only water.

2. Next add the sweetener to cups 2 through 5 as follows:
   Stir in ½ tablespoon corn syrup or sugar to the water in the second cup.
   Stir in 1 tablespoon corn syrup to the water in the third cup.
   Stir in 2 tablespoons corn syrup to the water in the fourth cup.
   Stir in 3 tablespoons corn syrup to the water in the fifth cup.

3. Testing: When you're ready, first take a sip of water from the reference cup. Then taste the sweetened water in the first cup and assess two things on the table below: its sweetness level on a scale from 1 to 10; and (yes or no) whether this level of sugar is intolerable (induces the gag reflex you get when you've had too much sugar). Write this value down on the table you create from the example we've provided.
   But before moving on to the next concentration of syrup, sip the cup of plain water to clear your taste buds. Then continue

on in that manner, making your way up the concentration gradient until you get to the last one, or until you get to the cup that's just too sweet for you.

A Tooth Table

SAMPLE TOOTH TABLE				
Week	½ tsp	1 tsp	2 tsp	3 tsp
1	3	5	7	8
2	4	6	9	X
3	4	5	8	X
4	5	6	9	X
5	5	7	X	X
6	6	8	X	X
7	7	X	X	X
8	8	X	X	X

Draw your own table to look like this one. For each sugar concentration, judge how sweet it tastes to you on a scale from 1 to 10, and then write it in the Week 1 row of boxes. If you get to the "gag me" level, where it's just too sweet to stand anymore, mark a big X in that box and those for all the stronger concentrations that follow it.

For the first week, test for your sweet tooth daily and average that number for the week. For the next weeks, test once per week on the same day each time, and write down the values. Keep in mind that your readings simply reflect the strength of your sweet tooth at that particular nanosecond. Even at that, you'll still be able to watch your taste for sugar drop over time. Remember, there's no absolute value that you should shoot for. In fact, the number you get when you do the test is completely arbitrary by itself. It only matters when you see how your sugar tolerance changes over time.

The Sweet Tooth Test reveals to you how quickly the values drop, as your cravings fade away.

What about sugar-free diet products? Won't they lower my sugar cravings?

Unfortunately, the answer is no. First of all, there are no diet soda bushes or roving herds of sugar-free fat-free puddings, ice creams, or Jell-Os out there. They do not exist outside of the chemical factory and the grocery store. Don't eat inventions.

Diet products actually drive up your sweet tooth even more than sugar! Your taste for sweetness is fed by foods that stimulate the sweet receptors on your tongue—sugar's only one of them. In fact, chemical sweeteners brag about how much sweeter than sugar they are, and so fuel your cravings for unhealthy oversweetened foods! Beyond the fact that chemical sweeteners are *all associated with health problems,* diet products defeat your efforts to tame the tooth.

Stealth Sugar Sources

It's been estimated that we eat an average of thirty-one teaspoons of sugars per day (Tufts University's Health & Nutrition Letter, June 2004). This may sound like enough to choke a horse, and it is, but think about this:

- A single twelve-ounce can of soda contains from nine to eleven teaspoons.
- Two ounces of hard candy can contain eleven teaspoons.
- One cup of Kellogg's Frosted Flakes cereal has more than four teaspoons.
- Sugar is hidden in a variety of forms: sucrose, invert sugar, maltose, maple syrup, glucose, dextrose, golden syrup, lactose, fructose, glucose syrup, brown sugar, fruit juices, sorbitol, mannitol, and zylitol.

Why Tame the Tooth?

I'm just going to pull from the huge databases at the National Institutes of Health regarding sugar consumption and show you what they say. Notice the rule that continues to resurface from the French approach. A little is beneficial. A lot is not.

CANCER: *"High intakes of sugar and refined carbohydrates and elevated blood glucose are strongly associated with the risk of cancer"* (Silvera, 2005).

SURVIVING CANCER: *"There is evidence that high carbohydrate intake is associated with poorer survival after diagnosis for early breast cancer"* (Krone, 2005).

CARDIOVASCULAR DISEASE: *"High blood glucose was associated with 1.8 to 3 times greater risk of death. The glycemic potential of carbohydrates is therefore relevant to both prevention and management of coronary disease"* (Brand-Miller, 2004).

KIDNEY STONES: *"It is concluded that consumption of cola causes unfavorable changes in the risk factors associated with calcium oxalate stone formation and that therefore patients should possibly avoid this soft drink in their efforts to increase their fluid intake"* (Rodgers, 1999; see also Weiss, 1992).

DIABETES: Dr. Willett from the Harvard School of Public Health has given us the skinny on sweetened beverages. *"Anyone who cares about their health or the health of their family would not consume these beverages."* And for good reason, too. Fifty-one thousand women examined over nine years in the Nurses' Health Study II showed an 80 percent increased risk of type 2 diabetes when they consumed either sugar or high-fructose corn syrup drinks. How much? As little as one soda or sweetened fruit drink per day. *One!* By the way, this was not the case for 100 percent fruit drinks.

OBESITY: Obviously too much sugar provides empty calories that lead to overweight, obesity, and diabetes, but think about the biggest sugar offender—high-fructose corn syrup. The problem with HFCS goes well beyond calories. As we've learned, this 100 percent fat-free sweetener doesn't clear from the blood like natural sugar, and so it stimulates the liver to make fat and triglycerides. This is but one good reason why you should avoid anything sweetened with HFCS.

Avoiding Added Sugar in the Real World

What about sugar you add to your drinks? First of all, don't worry about the extra twelve calories in a teaspoon of sugar. And especially don't think you have to resort to chemicals in your coffee or tea.

Try this. You know how the Sweet Tooth Test *reflects* your decreasing taste for sugary foods and drinks? Well, you can *cause* that to happen as well. You can drive down your taste for sugar in your drinks with a very simple experiment.

If you normally take three teaspoons of sugar in your drink, pull it back to two teaspoons for a week. I want you to assess how it tastes to you—especially at first. The lack of sugar will jump right out at you. But stick with the decrease for a while, and keep paying attention to this level of sweetness through the week. Soon it will seem perfect again and you'll have just changed what your body asks for. Congratulations!

If you want, you can eliminate all the sugar in your coffee—and still love it. You just have to give yourself time to adapt your tastes. This steady process is how you regain control over your desires and cravings. You don't have to choose unhealthy foods just because that's what you happen to like right now. This is truly a path. It's a journey from your current levels of food volume and food quality to a new, more productive level.

You get there by changing what you ask of your body. You stay there by changing what your body asks of you.

⚜ PEOPLE ON THE PATH

Dear Will,

By the time I began researching gastric bypass surgery, I was 5'3" and about 272 pounds. I have a small frame, so you can imagine how awkward and awful it felt to carry all that around. I was mentally exhausted from trying to lose weight and keep it off conventionally, and I wanted it to be over. So I had the surgery and, as predicted, off came lots of weight. If the story had ended there it would've been nice, but of course we know it didn't. I had no tools whatsoever to deal with the underlying cause of my eating, and felt like I was completely unable to cope.

When I came across your Web site and book, it was as if everything started to click at long last. I won't say that things became easier right

away, but I do like to think I listen to my inner voice and knew in-
stinctively when I learned about your philosophy that it was "right."

The area I feel most passionately about is regarding mindless, stress-
filled eating. Oddly enough (or not so oddly to you, I presume), when I
felt physically satisfied with what I'd eaten on your plan, it calmed me
down so I could think things through. That had been a huge problem
for me, the feeling of helplessness and panic that I might starve to
death. At that point I was able to see the things you had written for my-
self, like the newfound sweets craving was actually backward, that I
liked—or rather, needed—sweets only because I'd already been eating
them all along. The joy of a cup of tea with real half-and-half, and es-
pecially the satisfaction of it, can't be underestimated.

I want to tell you how much I appreciate your insight and advice
through this journey.

—Anne G.

Personal Responsibility

The most amazing piece of architecture I've ever had the privilege to
touch is the Pont du Gard near the southern French city of Nîmes. It's
a more than two-thousand-year-old Roman aqueduct with three levels
of arches spanning thirty miles, and crossing the Gardon River without
nails, rivets, or even mortar. Moreover, this stunning structure not only
still stands, but carried water flawlessly for five hundred years after the
fall of the Roman Empire.

As we moved across on the lowest level, seventy-six feet above the
river rocks below, I was amazed there was no fencing along the edge.
You could fall right off; you could lose a child. My lawsuit brain
screamed that this was a legal nightmare waiting to happen. After returning home, I asked a Lyon University law professor about this incredible liability. His answer surprised me.

"And who would you sue?" he challenged. "The bridge? It's been there for two thousand years." He started pacing, shaking his head. "If you were worried about the edge before you crossed the bridge, why did you climb on in the first place? And your children? If you let your kids fall off a bridge of two centuries, you are responsible, sir, not the state, not the city, and certainly not the Romans."

As I considered the obviousness of his viewpoint over the next few days, I realized the same should also go for our weight and health. We must assume a greater responsibility for our actions and stop pointing fingers at the causes of our problems. Many people want to retreat to blaming genetics, or carbs, or fats, or fast-food restaurants to explain their girth. But we have to take the wheel of control again and handle our own issues ourselves.

When you live this lifestyle with these healthy eating habits, you become empowered to handle your love handles yourself, by recognizing the reins you do have, right in your hands, and then taking charge of your situation. And your tool for accomplishing such a feat—sensual eating—is so delicious and awakening. You can do this, and you're going to love it in the process.

Sensual Eating: How to Taste

In *French Women Don't Get Fat,* Mireille Guiliano writes that the French don't have our weight problems because they eat with all their senses. The appearance, texture, taste, and aroma are all important. This sounds very good for enjoying your food, but how does sensual eating translate into weight control? It does so by being a very effective tool to help you eat small, slow down, and prevent overconsumption. You may have also heard the term *conscious eating,* which represents the same basic idea.

As you become more aware of taste, you'll subconsciously choose healthier foods. How many times have you found yourself mindlessly snacking on something you didn't even really like? This used to happen to me all the time with Big Gulp sodas so sweet they were dangerous, chocolates that tasted like wax, and chicken pressed into "nuggets." But as soon as you train your tastes to appreciate what you're putting in your mouth, the terrible quality of faux foods becomes obvious and you won't even want them anymore.

On the surface, it seems pretty simple—just take the time to pay attention to your senses. But it can actually be pretty challenging to remember to love your food in the hurry of a crazy day. The more you use these techniques, though, the better you'll be at them and the more they'll become a natural part of you.

Pleasure is a skill that you will cultivate by learning to appreciate the smell, texture, and flavor of your food.

Vision

One of the barriers you're going to find to sensual eating is actually vision. For example, when obese patients are blindfolded, they actually eat less food and appreciate it more. And even before you taste, notice the visual presentation. How ripe are the insides of the cut strawberries, how vibrant green is the steamed broccoli, and how golden is the pie crust? Notice. See what your food looks like before you actually eat it. You might even close your eyes when you're tasting something wonderful so you're not distracted by whatever you're looking at.

Flavor

Become aware of the salty tastes that blend into the savory flavors. Experiment with the way dark chocolate melts perfectly into the flavors of a rich red wine. Let the chocolate melt in your mouth, and taste the wine for a couple of seconds before you swallow it. Next, try a little dark chocolate with a dried cherry. It's fabulous. Notice how walnuts perfectly complement blue cheese (try a grape here, too!). And infuse your soups with ginger and experience how it completely lightens the flavor, as if you'd sprinkled it with the tart juice of summer lemons (see the recipe for Super Chicken Stock, page 290).

Aroma

Take note of the smell your food gives off in the pan and on your plate. Think about those aromas and try to pick out the ingredients they're coming from. Linger with the associations they carry: the warmth of onions chattering away in butter; the cozy fragrance of bread from the oven; the holiday excitement of cinnamon, nutmeg, and anything at all!

Texture

Feel the graininess of the Bosc pear in your mouth and notice the crisp coating of crème brûlée. The best textures are mixed, like truffles with their thin chocolate crisp of a shell surrounding a Chambord-infused ganache. Fresh bread's stiff crust and softer inner texture. Take small "tasting bites" so you can attend to the tactile nature of your food.

Over time you'll not only become better at sensual eating, but your palate will become sharper. So please don't worry if you really try, but can't quite tell the difference between mayonnaise and herbed mayonnaise, cheap chocolate and good chocolate, or cheese food and real cheese. You will.

Expect your senses to come alive over weeks, not days. This is another reason you don't want to waste a meal on faux food, because every time you do, you train your tastes in the wrong direction.

Don't Forget, Don't Diet

Freedom from dieting comes when you learn the life skills and healthy habits that control portions for you and increase the pleasure of eating while decreasing the volume at the same time. When you stop the diet mentality that frets over consuming x number of carbs or fats, you begin to taste—and love—your food again.

That skill of tasting has nothing to do with dieting, and everything to do with a lifestyle that naturally produces optimal weight, healthy hearts, and longer lives. That's because your taste buds come to recognize foods that are too overly sweetened, and they don't taste good to you anymore. You put that processed food in your mouth and realize that you don't even like the flavor.

And this is exactly why sensual eating is so important to the entire French approach. When you eat with your senses, you end up choosing higher-quality food, taking more time, eating smaller quantities, enjoying it more, consuming less, getting the health properties of the food without rampant overconsumption, and losing weight in the bargain. These are just the wonderful benefits of loving your food again. At that point you are not on a diet, but have reset your body's tastes for optimal health without even trying. Now you are in control, and naturally giving your body the healthful nutrients it needs. This is the key to low weight for life.

CHEAT SHEET: Sensual Eating and the Sweet Tooth

Taste and you become better at tasting. Not only do you awaken your senses to the flavors passing your lips, you also recognize how wonderful healthful foods are, and how unappetizing the faux foods are. Practice the art of sensual eating and soon you avoid harmful oversweetened foods because they just don't taste good anymore. And you choose healthful foods because you simply love the flavor.

Whenever you eat, take just a few minutes to think about the following:

- The level of sweetness
- How it looks on your plate
- The aroma your food gives off
- How certain flavors show up early, and others later
- The texture in your mouth

The Results You're Looking For
IMMEDIATELY
- You will notice food flavors and aromas and textures you never noticed before.
- You will understand how large your sweet tooth really is.

WITHIN TWO WEEKS

- You will notice that your sweet tooth becomes more sensitive.
- Sensual eating will become second nature.

WITHIN A MONTH

- You will choose foods low in sugar because that's what you love.
- Your habits of sensual eating will be refined and you will expand the education of your tastes.

HOMEWORK: TESTING YOUR TASTES AND PULLING THE TOOTH

1. Begin testing your sweet tooth daily for the first week.
2. Compare your first week's average to your measurements in later weeks.
3. Eat with your senses: notice the fragrance, texture, appearance, and taste of your food.
4. Practice eating with your eyes closed.
5. Judge the level of sweetness of ordinary foods.
6. Notice how sensitive you become to sugar levels over time.

PART TWO

How the French Eat

As the acknowledged gastronomic capital of France, Lyon is world famous for its thickets of traditional bouchon restaurants (*bouchon* literally means "wine cork"), as well as the brightest of cooking superstars, such as Paul Bocouse.

It's no wonder that the city with the best food in a country with the best food in the world spills more than one thousand restaurants onto its narrow cobblestone city streets. (Keep in mind that Lyon's population is only about 500,000 people.) Just over the left bank of the Saône, just beyond the weekend art exhibits and old men selling roasted chestnuts from a metal kettle drum, you'll find a nest of cafés and restaurants in the Old Lyon district. And there's no lack of patrons eating silky St. Marcellin cheese, fatty foie gras, and succulent crème brûlée!

Think about this for a minute. In America, we eat out more and more each year. In fact, our increase in energy consumption from restaurant foods has jumped a quantum 208 percent over the past twenty years. Experts quickly correlate the rise in "restaurant eating" itself to our escalating obesity rates. And yet in Lyon, a city known for rich food in the country known for rich food, there isn't an obesity problem, despite a love affair with restaurants that serve cream sauces, desserts to die for, and all the rest. How can that be?

The explanation isn't just about *what* the French are eating. We have to think a little more broadly. These thin healthy people can freely linger over luscious foods because of *how they're eating them!*

A meal in France is a delicious process that, if you're not familiar with it, can be quite a surprise. First of all, waiters aren't working for tips, so don't expect them to hurry you off your table . . . or hurry to serve you for that matter. Plus, no one expects you to blow in, eat in a rush, and run back out again. No one expects you to get your food "to go" so you can eat it at the red light!

It is *normale* to sit and enjoy your food for a while. In fact, in one of our first forays into the Lyon streets, our children pleaded with us to stop at a pizza restaurant with street-side seating. So we sat. We looked about, sat some more, and wondered if we were in the "do not serve" section. It must have been ten full minutes before the waiter showed up! Can you imagine? We entertained ourselves by people watching: couples were openly kissing on the streets (we weren't in Alabama anymore) and the diners around us were chatting away with food still on their plates, not in their mouths, or even in their hands. I wondered, *Don't these people have anything better to do than to sit around with their food all day?* Later I realized—maybe they're on to something.

Back home, if we ate for two hours—with our normal gulping habits—we'd plow through mountains of food and become gargantuan in no time. But, as I observed over and over, most French people don't eat how we eat. Their habits at the fork, the plate, and the meal are more different than most of us can imagine. Our motto is to "get in, get out, get on with your life"; I think theirs might be "get in, get settled, get on with your meal." But when you understand *how* they actually are eating, the paradox vanishes and you understand that their eating behaviors are what are making them thin.

But What About Genetics?

Could it be that the French physiology is just thinner because they have a population with "skinny genes"? And are we, by extension, overweight because we were programmed by our genes to be heavy? To answer this question, let's just look at the plain data.

One arcane academic trivia nugget produced by the Human Genome Project is the fact that the genetic difference between humans and the chimpanzee is only around 3 percent. Within our own species, population geneticists estimate that the genetic difference between us and our Neolithic ancestors is negligible. And yet, our obesity epidemic has exploded in the last thirty years (a genetic nanosecond). Therefore, whatever changed to cause this problem could not possibly be related to our genes. Since the global genetic makeup has not shifted in the past thirty years, it must be the environment: our food supply, eating habits, stress levels, activity levels. This is just plain, irrefutable logic.

So let's take a close look at the trends that have occurred as our obesity rates have been increasing. In a University of Miami paper entitled "The Macroeconomics of Obesity in the United States," Drs. Gomis-Porqueras and Peralta-Alva show that—since the 1960s—our expenditure on processed food products has increased 135 percent, and foods eaten away from the home have increased by 132 percent. Portion sizes? They have expanded to become two to five times greater than they were.

These trends show how our eating habits have changed. In the journal *Obesity Research*, Drs. Jeffery and Utter have shown more trends that have ushered in the obesity epidemic:

- From 1970 to 1994, we ate less butter by 13 percent, less whole milk, and drank more soda.
- We didn't buy our basic sustenance at food stores (which actually declined by 15 percent), but got it at ready-to-eat restaurants, snackbars, and vending machines, all of which more than doubled in this time period.
- The beneficiary of these trends was the processed food sector of the economy, which grew at a rate of 41 percent, right along with our obesity rate.
- From 1990 to 1998, the U.S. population actually increased its levels of exercise, and the number reporting "no physical activity" actually decreased.

Given these changes, our onset of obesity cannot logically be the predetermined result of our genes. The more obvious causes are these cultural changes that surround us. Our environment has become inundated with high-volume meals, fast-food eating, and faux foods. And all these changes have happened in lockstep with our growing obesity crisis.

If you believe your weight issues are genetic, you'll believe you are heavy by nature. You'll believe you can give up now—you might as well not even try. You could imagine this to be a mental refuge from the struggle of trying diet after diet and failing on them all. And because 90 percent of people fail on diets, you're in good company.

But the truth rests somewhere in the middle. Some things you can change and some you cannot. You can't think yourself taller or practice having a smaller bone structure. These are the cards you were dealt. On the other hand, if you dance you'll get better at dancing. If you type, you'll get better at typing. The question is not whether you can change your body, but where your windows of possibility lie. Where, exactly, can you train your body to adapt?

This entire section is a message of hope because it answers that question. There really is something you can do about your cravings, your chronic consumption, and the food choices that have led you into weight problems. You can change your behaviors to retrain your body to crave what is good for you. Once you learn these behaviors, you'll have them forever and can apply them for the rest of your life.

That's why the steps in this section are perhaps the most important part of *The French Don't Diet Plan,* because they give you the tools to learn how to eat for pleasure, even here at home. This series of steps begins when you relearn how to determine an appropriate bite. You then learn how to slow down so you can actually taste your food and appreciate what's in your mouth, develop a better relationship with delicious meals, and (as a happy side benefit) lose weight in the process.

After we learn to slow down, we'll solve portion distortion by redefining what it means to say, "I love my food." As you learn these new healthful eating habits, we'll also talk about *healthful drinking habits.* This isn't about alcohol, it's about the practice of controlling consumption across the board.

By the end of this section, you'll have all the tools you need from each step to achieve a lifetime of weight control automatically. You'll change not only your eating habits, but your entire relationship with food, and that's exactly what must happen in any long-term solution to weight management.

In the process you'll watch your body's expectations change in just days, see your cravings for junk foods go away, and feel your daily food dependencies fade. At the end of each step you can see the changes that will occur immediately, within two weeks, and even longer. This is all accomplished through what's known as your body's "appetite thermometer," the part of your brain that regulates hunger for your body just like your thermostat regulates temperature for your home. Turn down your appetite thermometer and you will *decrease how much you're hungry for.*

The end result? Learning the "how of eating" leaves you firmly in control of your body's cravings, rather than the other way around. This is the greatest freedom you could possibly experience and is the biggest missing piece to weight loss advice today.

Step ✤ 4

Spend More Time Enjoying Your Meal

Moments of culture shock happen when you step into the quirky mix of another environment. But they also hit you in reverse, after being away from home for a while and then coming back. By the time we returned from living in France, I'd become so accustomed to the leisurely pace of the French meal that I was in for a shock when I saw what I'd left behind.

My wife, Dottie, and I were at a nice restaurant with white linen tablecloths, candles, and flowers on the tables. After debating the menu choices, we finally ordered. As the waiter left us, we noticed a couple just sitting down at the next table. I glanced at them a few more times during our dinner.

By the time our main course arrived, they had ordered their meal.

By the time we were considering our dessert and coffee choices, they were done!

I thought something had gone wrong. Were they sick? Did they have an emergency? But a quick look at the table, and it was clear that they had just blown through a very nice dinner in about half an hour. I looked at Dottie and asked, "How do you even eat that fast?" How quickly I had forgotten that *we* used to eat that fast, too. This was the speed-eating cultural norm we'd both forgotten about, and one of the biggest factors fueling our incredible weight and health problems.

In this step, we'll talk about all the reasons this is true, and how to retrain your mind so you can slow down and control the size of your bites. This is critical because the faster you eat, the less you taste, and the more you consume to get that same sense of "flavor." They're all linked.

Dear Dr. Clower,

This approach has changed my life in so many wonderful ways. I appreciate food so much more now. I take the time to slow down and enjoy what I'm eating. And what I'm eating is amazing—no more deep-fried, partially hydrogenated, prepackaged, low-fat junk.

Real food. Fruit. Cheese. Bread. Butter. Fresh vegetables.

As a result, my skin is clearer, as is my thinking. My lifelong asthma has greatly improved, no doubt because I've stopped stuffing my body with chemicals.

I've always been pretty active, but my way of thinking about activity has changed for the better. Now exercise isn't something I do to punish myself, or to try to erase the effects of an overly large meal. It's not another "should" on my list. Instead, it's something I do for fun. For me. A nice walk after lunch, or some yoga stretches in the morning.

Weight loss was the reason I was drawn to the French approach in the first place. And while I've enjoyed that happy aspect of the program, it's truly been secondary to its greatest gift for me: learning to slow down and enjoy food—and enjoy life.

—Jennifer C.

Slowing Down

After spending one afternoon with a French colleague at a restaurant in our little hamlet of Meximieux, I must scientifically conclude that frog legs do, in fact, taste like chicken. They're sort of like buffalo wings of the sea. The texture is more tender, but the flavor is much the same.

Even though these delicate amphibian tenders were to die for, even though we were eating with our fingers, it still took about two hours for us to make it to the bottom of the plate. I was amazed—back home, I'd be done with a plate of wings in about ten minutes.

I realized it had been our friend Pierre who set the pace for the rest of us: eating a little, talking a little, and sipping crisp white wine before going back for the next frog leg. Unconsciously following his lead, we all ate in a leisurely manner.

However, the habits we learn eating with others often set the stage for speed-eating instead.

For example, have you ever seen someone eat with his or her arm around the plate? The person wraps such protection around it like a citadel, guarding the food fiefdom as if someone were likely to swoop down and scoop away his or her food, leaving our poor victim to starve to a slow, wilted death.

I've spoken to more than a few people who do this and they commonly say that, as kids, they trained themselves to protect their plates from siblings or parents who would snatch the occasional morsel. They laugh because they know it's a silly thing to do, but whenever they're not thinking about it, the arm shield comes back out to ward off all potential pillagers.

Speed-eating through our food has become a particularly common habit. Kids are given twenty-five minutes of lunch time, twenty minutes of which are spent in lines. Rushed parents grouse at kids who won't just hurry up and finish their food so they can get moving to something "important."

Think about how this frenzied eating pace is reinforced into adulthood, too. Lunch has become something to "work through," so you take enormous bites (bite-size has become defined as the amount you can fit in your mouth) so you can get through the meal faster. Even when your mouth is full, you have another bite on your fork or in your hands, at the ready, for the very moment when you can pack a bit more in your cheek pockets. And you flush your food down with your drink so you can gulp it back and get it over with.

This happens not just at a meal, but during an entire day. You wake up in the morning and rush through your breakfast (or eat it in the car), so you can zoom off to work with a thousand other rushing people, so you can hustle through your workday, so you can run home, blast through dinner, clean up, collapse in bed, and get up and do it all again the next day.

At every level, we have been trained to become a speed-eating nation.

So what, though? What's the problem with eating quickly? We absorb nutrients whether it takes two minutes or twenty to eat, right? Surprisingly, that reductionist view is just not true, and actually explains a major part of the French paradox.

Speed-eating is a 100 percent calorie-free eating habit that produces and sustains your long-term weight problems. In fact, a recent study by Britta Barkeling and her colleagues at Hudding University Hospital found differences in the way men of normal weight ate compared to those who were overweight. One of the most interesting differences was that "normal weight men typically took longer to eat, whereas obese men ate faster."

The same result was found for kids as well. "The eating behavior of 23 normal weight and 20 obese 11-year-old children was measured for the total intake of food, duration of consumption, and the relative rate of consumption. The obese children ate faster and did not slow down their eating rate towards the end of the meal as much as normal weight children."

Thus, a slower eating pace, like that innately practiced by the French, turns out to really matter for your weight and health. And the reason this so profoundly controls overeating has everything to do with the way your mind and body connect.

We typically think of feelings of fullness as being in our stomachs, because we sense them there. But this is not exactly the case. For example, say you get a paper cut on your finger. You look at it and say, "Ow, my finger hurts" (or some more colorful descriptive). But with just a little anesthetic, you could numb the nerve that runs along your arm and up to your brain. There would be a cut on your finger, but no pain. Therefore, the pain registers not in your finger, but in your head.

Likewise, you may stop eating when you feel like you've had enough in your stomach, but it's not your gut that's telling you that. It's your brain. To get those feelings of fullness into your brain, your body sends messages from many different sources (stomach, small intestine, and so on), through many different routes, such as nerves, and through chemicals released into the blood. And when they finally all drift into the brain, they get picked up over a scatter of neural centers, and have to get collated back into your subjective feeling that you're more or less full.

That's why satiety, if it were a painting, would be Impressionistic. Somehow all these different brain sites with all their different messages sent at different times to different locations sum up to equal "Whoa there partner, that's enough of them au gratin potatoes!"

The upshot of all this sprawling neurochemistry is this: There's a delay between being full and feeling full. It depends on your particular physiology, but it can take around fifteen minutes before those chemicals drift into your head so you begin to feel that you're satisfied with the meal. This simple fact is critical to controlling your consumption, and explaining why the French habit of slow eating helps make them thin. When you feel that familiar bowling-ball ache in your stomach after a meal, that's your signal that you've eaten too much too quickly. That uncomfortable feeling comes from the stretching of your stomach wall and happens whenever you take your body past "satisfied" and keep right on going into "stuffed."

Teenagers may be able to inhale a sandwich in less than a minute without gaining an ounce—I know mine can—but they are still immortal, omniscient, and have rapid metabolisms. In other words, a young person's physiology can get away with this immature eating style, but the rest of us cannot afford to. We face at least two problems when we speed-eat. The first is very basic and obvious. We're likely to take in too many calories at the meal and gain weight. But the second is even more important—we train our bodies to overconsume food in the long term.

Think of it like this: When you eat, there's an amount of food your body needs to live healthily. Let's say that, on a scale from 1 to 10, your body requires a level of 6. If you're eating hand over fist, rushing so you can get on to the next activity on your to-do list, at some point your body will have had enough (after it's gotten to a 6). But remember, it takes fifteen minutes before that full signal reaches your brain and you feel it.

Eating too quickly means that by the time those smoke signals manage to get up to your brain and say "Whoa there partner . . . ," you'll have put in a food level of 9! You'll have given your body much more than it ever needed and not only drastically overconsumed, *but conditioned your body to keep overconsuming.* If your body needs a level 6 of food today, but you give it a 9 . . . then tomorrow you give it a 9 . . . then the next day you give it a 9 . . . pretty soon it'll take 9 as the baseline volume of food it asks for. If you continue in this way, your body will soon be accustomed to consuming twice as much as you actually need. And this escalating portion distortion disaster happens simply by eating too much too fast.

Whether you're aware of it or not, you put your body in training with every act, every meal, every behavior. Practice doesn't make perfect, it makes permanent. Eat large, and large becomes normal for your body. Eat small, and small becomes normal. You decide what kind of eater you want to be, and then be that *on purpose* until your actions go from intentional (consciously performed) to automatic.

The good news is that, no matter where your baseline of hunger is right now, *you can move that level lower.* You can train your body to expect less food over time. And the very first step to regain control over your hunger is to practice taking your time with your meals.

So here's how to begin training your body in the right direction. Over your first week, extend the length of every meal—breakfast, lunch, and dinner—to at least twenty minutes. There are several techniques that can help make this happen. In the beginning, it might be helpful to set a countdown timer. Visualizing your food in quarters, allowing five minutes to finish the first quarter, five minutes for the second quarter, and so on, can be another very effective strategy.

Be sure to take note of your hunger level as you approach the end of your meal. This is the first step to becoming a "conscious eater" and paying attention to the sensations of satisfaction you get from eating. When you take just a minute to check in with your body as you go, you'll be far less likely to overdo it and far more likely to stop when you're satisfied to prevent overconsumption.

Finally, keep a notebook and write these observations down. They'll significantly change over time, and you'll be surprised at yourself even after the first few days have passed.

Coast into Feeling Satisfied

Timing, as they say, is everything. As you practice eating at a gracious pace, you'll realize just how much your satisfaction is delayed. So pause toward the end of a meal, and briefly to listen to your body. As you sit at the table and enjoy your friends, family, book, or music, *you'll notice that you're not satisfied yet.* Or that you're barely satisfied and really feel like you could eat another helping or so. But wait.

Be patient for just two to three more minutes and you'll feel those sensations coming on. You'll have added absolutely nothing more to your belly, but in only a minute or two you'll find that you're absolutely full.

Once you know this can happen to your body, it's the most amazing thing. You realize that you've actually had enough, but you just can't feel it yet. It's easy to see how this awareness of your own mind-body connection solves overconsumption for you, as you learn how to put on the brakes before overdoing it.

The solution is so easy and pleasant. Just relax at the table through your meal. Coast for a while after you're done and enjoy the people around you. This is the portion of the French meal where lingering conversation becomes an art. Even at the neurological hospital where I had lunch every day, the doctors and nurses with their busy schedules took their time at meals. I never saw anyone gulping down their last two bites of lemon tart or standing up to shove back their last bite of brie before their mad dash back to work!

The French, of course, don't adopt these slimming eating habits to control their weight. They practice them naturally because they love their food. But now you have to apply the French approach in your hectic life, in your own culture. Below are some of the pressures that may cause you to eat too fast, miss the flavor of your meals, and escalate your body's call for more and more food at the same time. Try the solutions that follow and you can make them work for you right away.

Situations That Make Us Eat Too Fast

❦ *Problem: Being in a hurry or distracted.*
   Solution: Stop before you start.

Focus on Your Food

"The eating rate was significantly slower among obese subjects when they ate blindfolded" (Barkeling, 2003).

This interesting study makes the point that, without the distraction of vision, subjects paid more attention to the smell, taste, and texture of the food, ate slower, and ate less of it. So attend to what you're eating and you'll slow your eating pace. Slowing down decreases consumption for you automatically.

A friend of mine runs one of the best Mediterranean markets in Pittsburgh. He came to me and groused that he had weight to lose. He eats the food he sells, so I know it's not only good, it's fabulous! I asked him how long it took him to eat his lunch, and he croaked "two minutes."

Ah. There you go. So I talked to him about sitting down and pacing his lunch, and how that one very simple eating habit—eating too quickly—was the source of his problems. I saw him six weeks later and he'd lost fifteen pounds.

Remember Physics 101? Objects in motion will stay in motion

until acted upon by an outside force. In this case, if you're living life at one hundred miles per hour, you're going to eat at that speed, too, overconsume, feel stuffed, and slide down the slippery weight-gain slope before you ever realize what happened. So insert a break to slow you down before you project that frenzy onto your lunch or dinner.

- *Say a prayer or meditate.* When I was growing up in Alabama, it was a given that everybody prayed before a meal. Now that I'm out on the open globe, I see people doing the same basic thing by giving a quick nod of thanks to the universe or just relaxing for a minute before beginning dinner. The French generally don't pray, but they do pause before starting their meals. This practice gives them time to mentally unwind and relax a bit first.

  However you choose to plug it into your personal cosmology, the result is the same. Just listen to this research result from Dr. Barkeling: "A higher initial eating rate reflecting eating drive was associated with signs of stress overload. . . . The stress overload may prompt eating, and affective responsiveness may be linked to appetite through a higher sensitivity to food stimuli, thus increasing eating drive. An accelerating rate of consumption during the meal was associated with intense emotionality and oral dependency."

  Here's the science-to-English translation: Relax in some way before you start eating or you'll eat too fast. Eat too fast and you'll eat too much. Eat too much and you'll lose control of your weight and health.

- *Take a few deep breaths* (see Step 9 for more on these mini-meditations). If you find yourself hurried into a meal, the best you can do for yourself is to close your eyes, take a few lingering breaths from your belly, and then start. This calms you down so you don't apply the pace of your rapid-fire life to your meal.

  Remember, everything has its own inertia, or momentum, including you. That's why rule number one to make the French approach work in your life is to give yourself the freedom to take your time with your meal. Then you can enjoy it without overeating.

⚜ *Problem: Passive overconsumption.*
Solution: Focus on your food.

If you're distracted by something (eating in the car, watching TV, walking back to your job), you're likely to overeat. It's that simple. Dr. Jennifer Utter and colleagues, reporting in the *Journal of the American Dietetic Association,* are among the groups of scientists showing that "television/video use among boys and girls [is] associated with more unhealthful dietary behaviors (e.g., increased consumption of soft drinks, fried foods, and snacks)."

The science is very clear about this phenomenon. Writes Brigitte Boon in a 2002 study, "As predicted, . . . restrained eaters ate the same amount as unrestrained eaters when not distracted, but considerably more when distracted. There was also an unexpected main effect, which indicated that [all] eaters ate more if distracted than if not distracted."

The science-to-English translation? Pay attention to what you're eating. You'll taste more if it and eat less of it.

Research aside, just think about this intuitively for a minute. If you don't even notice what you're putting in your mouth because you're dodging traffic or focused on something far more pressing (like *Seinfeld* reruns), you'll just keep putting hand to mouth.

The French solution to this problem is so easy to apply. First, here are the don'ts: Don't eat in the car if you can help it. Don't eat while watching TV if you can help it. Never eat on your feet. The French don't even have drink holders in their cars! They could not imagine eating while walking back to the office, as if the meal were no more important than blowing your nose or running an errand.

Now the dos: Do return to the family table (see Step 8). Do eat with people you enjoy being around and make time to include them. Do set the table. Do practice sensual eating and focus on how good your food tastes instead of some other activity. And finally, do set aside your eating time and make it a priority in your day.

❧ *Problem: Keeping your food in your hand.*

Tonight, when you eat, try this experiment. As you're chewing a bite, look at your hand. Is there a forkful of food in it? Are you waiting for the very second when you can slip more food in your mouth? Realize that the only, only reason to still have food on your fork or in your hand is to get more in your mouth. This seemingly benign but insidious habit can be one of the most difficult ones to break, but it must be broken because it absolutely makes you eat too much too fast.

Solution 1: Establish a healthy rhythm of eating.

If there's food in your mouth, there should be nothing poised on your fork, waiting like a plane on the runway. Here's the rule: If food's in your mouth, nothing's in your hand.

As you spend your leisurely twenty minutes at a meal, practice this healthy eating routine:

- Take a bite-size piece.
- Put your food or fork down.
- Completely finish what you have in your mouth.
- Only then pick up your food or fork.
- Have another bite-size piece.

This habit won't serve you well until it gets worn into a comfortable groove by repetition. So, to make this rhythm a natural part of your relationship with food, begin by mentally reminding yourself of this new pacing routine until it becomes second nature. If you find that you have to think about it to make it happen, don't worry. Soon you'll look down and see that you've set your fork down subconsciously. That's the goal!

Solution 2: Engage in conversation.

If, as they say, hunger is the best sauce, then conversation comes in a close second. It's the most pleasant part of the meal and a normal part of the French table. Remember conversation? That's what we used to do before eating became a point between errands. And it needs to be revived because talking at the table with your friends is actually a wonderful weight loss strategy.

If you're enjoying a conversation with friends or family, you're not eating nonstop. This alone can slow you down enough to let the satiety signal drift up to your brain, so you can feel when you've had enough. And when you're in animated conversation, you tend to talk with your hands—so they're not picking up food!

So first be sure to take small bites and pause long enough between them to be able to say something without your food spilling out. When you think about the course of your meal, aim to have as much time with your mouth empty as full. And the perfect way to do this is to introduce conversation into the mix.

If you're dining alone, read something you enjoy during dinner or listen to music. This also slows you down so you can enjoy your food more, and eat less in the process. The key for you will be setting the fork or food down between bites. Since you don't have a companion to bounce thoughts off, you'll lean more heavily on the healthy rhythm of eating above.

❧ *Problem: Taking bites that are way too big.*

If you tend to fill your fork and mouth to capacity and gulp down your meal, you'll be done in no time. Are you getting a visual? If this is you, chances are your sense of bite-size is way off and needs to be retrained, or you'll keep overeating at this most basic level. Bite size, like the size of our plates and servings and drinks, has blown through the roof in the last few years. The volume knob has been cranked up on everything we eat, including our sense of what a bite actually is.

If you want your changes in eating behavior to last, start with a strong foundation. And the very first change is with your bite, with a rule of thumb you can follow every day. Something simple and intuitive with a size measure you can carry with you all the time.

Solution 1: Use the "rule of thumb," a bite-size exercise.

Hold up your hand in front of you, palm facing toward you. Give yourself the thumbs-up sign with that hand. Now bend your thumb's top joint down.

Next, I want you to lightly touch your teeth to the top and bottom of your bent thumb (lengthwise, from knuckle to tip). Then, without changing the size of your open mouth, take your thumb out and notice how wide your mouth is.

It's huge! You should never take a bite larger than this. Try the same exercise by turning your thumb sideways. Even at this, your mouth is plenty big.

Now take a look at the top segment of your thumb. Admit it. It looks like a nano-nibble at best, and there's no way it could possibly be enough for a bite. But when you do this objective test, and think about how big you'd have to stretch your mouth open to get anything larger in there, you realize that it's about right.

VITAL STATS ON A THUMB JOINT: 1¼ inches long, ¾ inch wide.

This is part of the problem, isn't it? Our perception of food quantity has become enlarged, like seeing it through a warped circus mirror. We've got to flatten that mirror and finally return ourselves to a realistic judgment.

So use the rule of thumb as the maximum bite size for the food you put in your mouth. If it seems like cruel and unusual punishment to eat that small, it's only because you've become accustomed to normally huge bites. But it actually doesn't take more than a couple of weeks until your thumb-size bites seem perfectly normal. Moreover, this very easy and intuitive rule can be used when eating with silverware or with your fingers.

Solution 2: Use the right tool for the right job.

The rule of thumb is helpful but, much of the time, your bite size is determined by the dimensions of your fork or spoon. The larger the spade, the more fill you'll put on it. If you run into this problem, there's a simple solution. Eat with a dessert fork or small spoon.

VITAL STATS ON A DESSERT FORK: 1½ inches long, 1 inch wide.

Keep in mind that you're likely to experience the same initial psychological response, and think that this baby fork is ridiculously tiny! But "large" and "small" are only meaningful in relation to other things. If it seems little to you, then you know you've been eating too large all this time. But you can change your own sense of large and small by making these simple changes.

And that's the best part. You get to decide. You're in control.

I don't think anybody wants to overconsume—it just happens unconsciously when your habits cause you to eat so large. That becomes your norm. But you really *can* be a small eater! Just use the rule of thumb with every bite until it becomes natural.

Solution 3: Become a people watcher.

When you go to a restaurant, observe how thin people eat. Just take note. Then watch how overweight people eat. Again, compare those habits to your own. Even after you've already ordered your food, you'll notice people who enter the restaurant, wolf down their meals, and then leave before you do. You'll notice people who stuff their mouths and themselves. You'll see people gobbling through their meals and never speaking to one another.

They're not tasting their food, they're just inhaling it. When you see that and realize how bad it is, you begin to identify the destructive eating habits as those you don't want to have for yourself—and the healthy eating habits as those you do want. That identification is a wonderful training tool. Do this every time you eat and you'll be less likely to replay their mistakes—and more likely to adopt the others' healthy habits.

Solution 4: Guesstimate when you eat with your hands.

Managing your bite size with your fork is easy. Just cut the food into realistic little pieces. Then you actually see the size and can make sure you're following the rule of thumb. But what do you do when you have a slice of pizza or your morning *pain au chocolat?* You could cut them, but it's more likely that you'll just eat them by hand.

This is why finger foods and convenience foods can quickly sabotage your weight loss efforts. It's so easy to pick up five fries at a time, fill up your cheek pouch, and drive on. It's much more difficult to estimate a normal bite size with a pizza slice. So you have to judge the rule of thumb on the fly, and take no more than an inch of that pizza or hamburger or fry at a time. Most of us have trouble with this estimation so, at first anyway, try slicing your food into the appropriate size.

This is where bite size is really going to hit you. The first time you cut off one inch of that wedge, you'll think, "Wow, that's tiny!" But this reaction simply means that you're relearning the bite size that will help take your weight off, not put it on.

The second rule for handheld food is the same as the rule for eating with a fork—but it's even more important for handheld foods. *If you have food in your mouth, get the food out of your hands.* Set the pizza, croissant, or sandwich down. Don't worry, it's not going anywhere. No one's going to rush in and snatch it away from you.

It matters even more to set handheld foods down because of the neurological connection between your mouth and your hands. Have you ever watched people perform something difficult or complex with their fingers? Contortions seize their mouths, as their lips curl and their tongues snake around their teeth. It's funny to watch, and reflects the strong neural link we all have between the hands and mouth.

Thus, as long as you're holding something tasty, your natural oral fixation lures it right into your mouth. And that gravitation is even greater when you're distracted by TV, driving, or when you're eating on your feet. Whenever your mind is on something else, automatic reflexes kick in to put food to mouth. Short-circuit them by simply setting your food down.

Don't Forget, Don't Diet

Why doesn't a five-minute Slim-Fast shake, or a two-minute low-carb breakfast bar work in the long run as a weight loss tool? As we see with the French approach, it's because basic habits of healthy weight loss work from the bottom up. Controlling your *pace* is a far more effective tool to control your portions (as we'll see in the next step), which permanently controls your weight. Small changes cascade into long-lasting results.

As you take your time and coast into feeling satisfied after the meal, the volume of food you consume will drop, the meal becomes enjoyable again as you spend more time talking to family and friends, and you lose your fear of fats, carbs, and proteins. You become more aware of your body's satiety signals, and understand when you should stop eating. Finally, that uncomfortable stuffed feeling will never happen again.

But this is a process, and it takes time. If you forget your new eating behaviors and find yourself stuffed after a meal, don't worry. Just look back and note that you ate too much too fast, and resolve to reinforce your habits at the next meal so you can stop when you're satisfied that time. And it's just this kind of ongoing training that instills the lifetime behaviors that produce low weight for life.

No more dieting, no more deprivation, because you no longer need them.

CHEAT SHEET: Take Your Time

Taste your food by eating small and eating slowly. Remember that any new skill starts in your head before sifting down into your hands. In other words, you'll have to make these lessons happen *on purpose,* by simple practice, so they can become second nature.

Practice makes permanent.
Control your pace, to control your portions, to control your weight.

Loving Your Food
- Take at least twenty minutes to eat your meal.
- Pace yourself at the table to control portions automatically.

- Enjoy meals with friends.
- Size matters! Use the rule of thumb to determine your bite size.
- If you have food in your mouth, set the food, fork, spork, spoon, cup, or bowl down, so it's not in your hand.
- Relax. After your meal, wait for the feeling of satisfaction to catch up with you.

The Results You're Looking For

IMMEDIATELY

- You'll never be stuffed again.

WITHIN A WEEK

- The volume of food you consume at a meal will drop.
- Meals will become enjoyable again, because you'll spend more time talking to family and friends, and less time eating.

WITHIN A MONTH

- You'll learn these new habits so well that you don't even have to think about them, and your weight loss will follow.

Step ⚜ 5

Plan on Seconds

Have you ever lived in a location that had some wonderful attraction, but you never managed to go until you had guests that you had to "show around"? Fortunately for us, when we lived in France we probably had three weeks during our entire stay in which we did not have visitors. So we developed some standard routes for showing them around the various sites and scenes.

One of my favorites was the Lyon morning market, followed by a mid-morning walk up the hill to the beautiful Fourviere Cathedral. And after all that exercise, we just had to finish up by taking our guests to any of the restaurants to eat. By the time we'd stroll back to the right bank of the Saône across the Marèchal Juin bridge, the market had folded up, moved on, and the restaurant district of Presque'ile (almost an island) awaited—just one short block in and a quick dodge to the left.

Typically, for our guests, some things were instantly recognizable: the Old World, cobblestone streets, rows of restaurants with the clatter of outdoor tables, waiters flaunting their superior air, and the aura of fabulous food all around. But the menus were another matter altogether. After getting seated and translating the dishes for them—being careful to highlight which were the "Lyonnaise specialty" internal organs—we would point out that the French typically eat in courses: an appetizer perhaps, followed by the entree, salad, dessert, cheese, and coffee.

One very weight-conscious friend's eyes widened at this, with her "Oh MY God" expression. "That's going to be a ton of food!" I tried to tell her that she didn't have to eat it all, but she assured me that yes, once it arrived on the plate, she probably did.

Her biggest surprise was that indeed we ate for almost an hour and a half and, by the end of the meal, she didn't feel stuffed.

Each French course is sumptuous, but small, too. And, because you know you've got more rich food coming, you don't really mind the size. After all, you're not expected to fill up completely on the first, second, or even third course. Thus, these multi-course meals have nothing to do with how much you can "put away." They're all about enjoying each course as it comes out—and you can't do that if you're stuffed after the first one! Think of it as "serial tasting."

I'm going to show you how to make this everyday French habit work for you, even when you aren't able to have a multiple-course dinner. But you should first know the two biggest issues that we have to overcome to apply these wonderful habits: confusing quantity with quality and conflating the love of food with simple gluttony.

The Difference Between Love and Gluttony

"The French truly love their food, and that's why they don't overconsume." Doesn't that sound wrong? I was speaking by phone with a U.S. health reporter and pointed out that the French are thin *because they really love their food*. She stammered, "Wait. Don't we have horrible weight and health problems precisely because we love our food too much?"

That view is very common, and actually represents a huge cause of our weight problems. We've confused the love of food with gluttony. This cultural misconception about food is laced throughout our basic behaviors. For example, when people say they love their food, they demonstrate it by eating large volumes, very quickly. Conversely, if you see someone take small bites and eat slowly, you naturally assume that they don't really like it. Think about what this cultural assumption means for us: Love has been reduced to consumption.

This belief is so ingrained in our subconscious that we don't even realize what's going on, why it's harmful, or the impact it has on our weight problems.

By contrast, the French don't think of loving food as an exercise in ravenous consumption. They don't even have an expression similar to "pig out." Rather, for them it's more about the sensual experience of enjoying delicious food. They treat their love of food like any healthy relationship. In essence, all of the things that make the food wonderful have the French diner's attention when they're eating, rather than the TV, the traffic situation, or the computer screen.

For our part, if we were to love a person like we "love" our food, we'd call that a disturbed relationship. If you just had to have a person, but hated yourself for that behavior every bit as much as we feel guilty for wanting wonderful foods, we'd send you to counseling. If you had to be around them, but treated them as an incidental bother or errand less important than reruns, phone calls, and schedules, we'd realize that eventually someone's going to get hurt.

In any relationship, the confusion between love and consumption is corrosive.

Confusing Quantity with Quality

For thirty-nine cents extra, fast-food restaurants and all-you-can-eat buffets tell us we can have twice the volume of food and a bucket of soda to wash it back with. This marvelous marketing ploy works because our beliefs have been conditioned to two-dimensional mathematics. Volume equals value. Quantity equals quality. And it's not just food. This idea appears in all our choices—from homes to Hummers—that conflate worth with size.

A while back, a commercial for a hamburger company featured a kid holding a burger. You could see that he was very excited about this sandwich and was getting ready to lay into it. When he started eating, the film sped up. Zip zip zip, he's done. Then he inhaled with a smile on his face and let out a noisy satisfied exhale.

Marketers spend millions of dollars to figure out what you believe so they can give it to you attached to their wrapper and icon. They gave you this kind of commercial on purpose. Why? Because loving your food, for us, means that you eat it big, and eat it fast.

When these equations are applied to dinner, normally healthful foods become unhealthful, because most people believe that healthful foods and unhealthful foods are different items. But the confusion between love and gluttony, quantity and quality, makes this completely untrue. We've got to understand this most basic principle.

Here's a simple example. If your doctor gave you a prescription and told you that one pill per day was going to make you feel better, would you take the whole bottle because you wanted to feel *really good*? Of course not. Even though a little is good for you, several times the dose of the very same pill can kill you. The beneficial nature of the medicine is not just about that bottle of pills, *but also how you consume them*. If someone dies of an overdose, it's not because of the medicine, it's because they abused the medicine.

The same principle is just as valid for foods and beverages. Wine and butter are perfect examples: One to two glasses of wine per day is very good for your heart, but one to two bottles per day is terrible for your liver. Butter has vitamins A and E, as well as selenium, which are very good for you, but if you eat a bucket of butter, it will choke your arteries.

Thus, food and drink are not the enemy. Overconsumption is. That's because there's nothing you cannot kill yourself with by simply having too much of it. This central issue has been the single greatest contributor to our weight and health problems as we've cycled through low-fat and low-carb diets. All through these fads, everyone has assumed that, if you just control the molecules, you can eat more and more of the food.

This is a complete fallacy—even when the food's low-fat! Danish researcher Jeppe Matthiessen summarized this point straight from his

research: "Larger portion sizes of foods low in fat . . . could be important factors in maintaining a high energy intake, causing overconsumption and enhancing the prevalence of obesity in the population.
In light of this development, portion size ought to take central place in
dietary guidelines and public campaigns."

You do the math. Low-fat products plus high volume eating equals
overconsumption, overweight, and obesity.

Luckily, there is a simple rule you can use to control your eating
volume so that wonderful real foods such as chocolate, wine, butter,
and eggs remain as healthful as they've always been. Love your food.
This simple lesson explains the paradox that the French can eat high-
fat and high-carb foods every day and yet don't have our weight and
health problems. They keep their foods healthful by having better relationships with them. Here's how to love your food again:

- To love your food, really, means to spend more time with it, not
  less. When I'm traveling on tour, I'm consistently approached by
  people who tell me that they or some member of their family
  lingers longest with their food and they're the skinniest ones in
  the bunch. And they're thin for all the reasons we've said. Eating
  at a relaxed pace just means you spend more time with less food
  overall.

- To love your food, really, means judging it by your palate, not your
  wallet. It's about the visual appeal, the aromas that fill your
  home, and the flavor and savor you get bite by delicious bite.
  Food is not good because its size approximates that of your head
  or because you paid only ninety-nine cents for it. In fact, "value"
  foods are cheap only because they're made with cheap materials.

- To love your food, really, means actually tasting it. Why be a
  mindless eater? Use all your senses so you can appreciate what
  you have. With smaller bites, you're more apt to notice the
  flavors, aromas, and texture, thereby enjoying it more and eating
  less in the process.

So love your food again! That's what this entire approach is all about.

✤ PEOPLE ON THE PATH

Dear Will,

I started this way of eating on May 15, 2004. I have lost twenty-five pounds since then, steadily, and I still seem to be losing. I cannot emphasize enough how much food has become a complete nonissue. Well, in a way. I don't have a constant sense of shame in my thoughts and behaviors in relation to food. It's like that emotional baggage just dropped away. I can't remember the last time I thought, "Oh, my God, I shouldn't eat this. I'm going to get fat. I'm too fat already. Yada, yada, yada." I just eat what I want and don't give it a second thought. No chemicals though. That's the only thought I give it.

In another way, it's become a guilt-free, delicious focus. I use whole milk, butter, cheese, olive oil, veggies, fruits, homemade bread, chocolate, all these things that are "sinful." I'm enjoying cooking not only as a creative outlet, but as a serious addition to my health.

Not only has my eating changed, but my SPENDING has changed. I'm not buying that fake garbage at the grocery store anymore. In fact, besides toilet paper and soap, my local farmers' market gets ALL of my money. So I guess I'm happy about what you're doing, I support you, and if there's anything that I can do to help, please let me know.

Sincerely,
Julie B.

Curing Portion Distortion

Put food in front of a goldfish and it'll eat it. Put a lot of food in front of a goldfish, and it'll eat it all. In fact, it'll eat until it hurts itself.

And yet, are we so different?

- More goldfish die every year of overfeeding than of any other cause.
- Obesity now closes in on tobacco as the number one preventable cause of death.

Why do we eat too much? It sounds obvious, but one biggie-size reason is because (like goldfish) we just don't know when to stop. Unfortunately, if there's food in front of us, we'll swim on over and gulp it down until it's gone.

Portions are too large, so people eat too much. But aside from the fact that eating too much nets you too many calories at the plate, worse is that this extra food has no bearing whatsoever on how much you're going to eat at the next meal! When Dr. Tanja Kral gave test subjects larger portions at one meal, she and her Penn State colleagues found that "subjects did not compensate for the additional intake by eating less at the subsequent meal. The findings indicate that large portions of foods . . . facilitate the overconsumption of energy." In other words, a big lunch doesn't mean you'll have a small dinner. It just means you'll have too much to eat!

For all these reasons, we must retrain our minds to think completely differently about our servings. If you want to eat healthy again, you must eat small and cure your portion distortion. The prior step covered the strategies we can use for forks and fingers, but there's plenty more work to be done at the plate as well.

Smaller Plates

"Bottomless Bowls: Why Visual Cues of Portion Size May Influence Intake": This is the title of the 2005 research by obesity scientist Dr. Brian Wansink and his colleagues, who performed a clever study. They compared how much soup two groups of subjects consumed until they were full. The first group ate from normal-size bowls. The second group ate from modified bowls that slowly, imperceptibly, refilled themselves.

Both groups ate until the soup was finally gone, but the "bottomless bowlers" ate a whopping 73 percent more than the others. The interesting part of this tale is that the participants who ate so much more didn't even notice. Incredibly, writes Dr. Wansink, "they did not believe they had consumed more, nor did they perceive themselves as more sated than those eating from normal bowls."

Eating was not based on the sensation of fullness, and subjects stopped spooning in the soup only when they saw that their bowls were finally empty. This is a prime example for the lesson we stress throughout this book. Your subjective sensations of hunger do not necessarily mirror your physiological need for food. Again, from Dr. Wansink: "It seems that people use their eyes to count calories and not their stomachs." In this case, subjects had eaten all they needed, but the power of the visual stimulus (soup still left in the bowl) overrode any other signals, and they just kept eating.

Thus, eating more does not make you more satisfied. It just makes you eat more.

Portion Control and the Mind-Body Connection

Physiologically, your body has a variety of sensors to clue you in that you're hungry for a certain amount of food. But that need for food must reach consciousness for you to be aware of it (aka your feeling of hunger). And the translation between your body's need and your mind's interpretation of that need is definitely not direct.

In other words, your mind amplifies your body's signal. You may feel ravenous, like you could literally eat everything on the menu, but that's not actually true. Your mind overestimates what your body needs. This translation error makes all kinds of biological sense. The safest possible survival strategy would be to generate an urgency far in excess of the actual need. This would make sure you got out there to score enough food to prevent any chance of starvation. If you're Joe Hunter-Gatherer, this is a smart solution.

But today, our modern overabundance is not appropriate for our instincts anymore. Welcome to weight problems. The solution is to compensate for the urges that have now become out of place. Because your mind overestimates your body's needs, we should underestimate our urges. That way we'll hit it just about right.

This portion control solution begins with scaling down the size of the plate itself. Use medium-size plates instead of large ones. The hardest part of this will be when family celebrations come around and you're used to serving everyone on platters. But remember, especially when you begin on this lifestyle, the amount in front of you determines the amount you will eat.

Understanding that basic fact is exactly how you begin to regain control over your food and weight. It starts with a decision on your part to order small and serve small. That way, *you get to decide* if you overeat or not. Start small and you'll end small. This is easy!

But what if you're ordering out? Let's take pizza as the perfect example. If you order a pizza and set the box on your lap in front of the TV, the box becomes your plate, and your body will think of the entire pizza as a *portion*. The solution is that, when it arrives, serve a slice on a plate and set the box in the oven on a low temperature to keep it warm. Only serve yourself one piece at a time. You can always go back if you want more, but this way you prevent the mindless gobbling that a lapful of pizza can produce.

Your Guide to Proper Portions

Remember that these portions are approximate and your own amounts will change over time. But, as suggestions, they provide a good reference point.

Drinks don't count as a portion, as long as they're in the small category (six ounces or so). If your drink is larger than that, it counts as one portion. All drinks must be "real"—water, tea, coffee, wine, juice, and not diet or regular sodas (see Step 3 for information on their effects on you).

BREADS
   1 slice whole-wheat, rye, white, or pumpernickel bread
   ½ English muffin

½ bagel

1 dinner roll

One 6-inch-diameter pita bread

One 6-inch-diameter corn or flour tortilla

CEREALS AND GRAINS

1 cup cold cereal

1½ cups puffed cereal (for example, puffed rice)

½ cup cooked cereal (for example, oatmeal, oat bran, cream of wheat)

½ cup cooked brown or white rice

½ cup cooked pasta or soba noodles

SNACK FOODS

1 ounce cheese (think of four dice)

1½ cups popped natural popcorn

2 tablespoons crunchy peanut butter or hummus

4 to 6 whole-wheat crackers

Two 4-inch-diameter rice or corn cakes

6 unsalted nuts (such as Brazil nuts)

6 large black or green olives

4 slices Melba toast

VEGETABLES (THINK OF A RACQUET BALL)

½ cup cooked or canned beans, lentils, or peas (lima, kidney, black, and so on)

½ avocado

1 cup raw leafy vegetables (for example, kale, spinach, romaine, arugula, bibb lettuce, iceberg lettuce, and watercress)

1 cup raw vegetables (for example, carrots, broccoli, asparagus, and onions)

½ cup cooked vegetables (most kinds)

1 small, 3-ounce baked potato

½ cup cooked mashed potatoes

FRUITS (THINK OF A TENNIS BALL)

1 small, 4-ounce apple

½ cup applesauce, unsweetened

1 medium banana

¾ cup berries or melon

1 medium peach, nectarine, kiwi, or plum

½ medium grapefruit

½ cup fruit cocktail, in its own juice, without syrup

4 prunes (also called "dried plums")

2 tablespoons raisins or other dried fruit

MEATS (THINK OF A PACK OF PLAYING CARDS)

⅓ pound chicken, turkey, fish, beef, or pork

2 slices bacon

1 can fish such as herring or sardines

1 small can tuna in water

DAIRY (THINK OF FOUR DICE)

1 ounce most cheeses (Parmesan, mozzarella, ricotta, and so on)

2 eggs

8 ounces (1 cup) milk or variants

4 ounces (½ cup) plain or fruit yogurt

1 to 2 tablespoons butter

2 tablespoons cream, half-and-half, or sour cream

Plan on Seconds

I know you can't always eat in courses (realistically, we don't all have time to make appetizers, soup, and salad to go with the main dish), but you can still make this principle work for your weight and health.

So, dinner's ready, you've got a spoon in the peas, and everyone in your family has their smaller plates outstretched to be served. Now what? How do you control food volume? How much should you scoop out onto the plates? The answer is very simple: Plan on seconds.

I love this rule because, like the one that says we should love our food *more,* something about it sounds so wrong. People hear this and think

I'm advising them to gobble even more, when in fact it results in just the opposite effect. Planning on seconds actually causes you to eat less.

It works like this: There's no need to measure out food quantities on a scale. When you have food to dole out on your (medium-size) plate, serve yourself an amount small enough so that you'll look at it and think, "That's *not quite enough* for me. I'm going to have to go back for seconds." That amount is your perfect portion.

By planning ahead of time to go back for seconds, you set yourself up for success, not failure. Now use the habits of healthy eating learned in the prior step, and take your time with that amount over twenty minutes. When you finish the food on the plate, you'll find that most of the time you're perfectly satisfied with your original portion. (Be prepared to "coast" into satisfied. See Step 4.)

If after twenty minutes you are not content, and you need a bit more, apply the same rule to plan on (in this case) thirds. Put an amount on your plate that you think isn't quite enough, even if that's just a bite or two. Then take your time with your seconds until you're done. By this time, you should feel satisfied. If not, consider having dessert. Yes! You get to have dessert!

Do the very same thing when you eat in courses. Have them in small manageable increments, each of which is less than the total amount you're hungry for. Consciously avoiding a single huge plate of food will train your body to not overeat. By the way, this is not about fooling yourself with a visual trick. It's an intelligent way to take advantage of the way your body's physiology of hunger operates.

❧ Problem: "Clean Your Plate."

The equation below is the scientific validation of something we all know as the clean-your-plate problem. Its basic math runs like this: There are starving children in third-world countries plus food stares up at you from your plate equals keep eating until it's gone. We've already covered the basic solutions to this common parentally induced problem—start with a smaller plate and plan on seconds—but now we're going to add homework for you to practice.

Solution 1: Leave food on your plate.

- We shouldn't eat just because food is within reach, we should eat because we're hungry.

- We don't stop eating just because there's no more food in sight, we stop when we're full. But to know when to stop and start, to even be able to hear your body's signals, you must be comfortable with having food left in front of you, *and with not eating it when you're not hungry.* This is a skill that you must practice just as you would any other task.

Learn to be at peace with leaving food on your plate. The amount you leave doesn't matter, as long as you keep at it. When you clean up, you have permission to toss those last four macaroni noodles or carrot pieces in the trash—or into a Tupperware container if you like. It's a good exercise. And the more you do this the better you'll become at it. The control and confidence you get from mastering this situation will apply across situations: the cookie jar, the holiday junk fest at the office, and between-meal munchies.

Solution 2: Plan on dessert.

When you live this lifestyle, you can have dessert after any meal—but only if you aren't satisfied yet. If you've eaten enough at dinner and are nicely content, you might not have dessert. You've already given your body its fill, and dessert will just pile on more where it's not needed or wanted.

Prepare for dessert by planning on it—and finishing dinner without being full already. Think about this as a wonderful preparation for what lies ahead. And whatever dessert you're having will taste so much better if you're not already full!

At home, we typically wait for ten to fifteen minutes before having dessert. We'll sit for a while or pick up the plates and put away the food, and then put out the pie or serve the ice cream or whatever it is.

When you do have dessert, treat it just like you do your food. Take small bites, put your fork or spoon down between bites, and make it last long enough to really enjoy it.

Don't Forget, Don't Diet

Prescriptive diets will tell you, to the gram, how much you should portion out for yourself. You're under the constant scrutiny of carb counters or fat counters or point counters. What's the problem with this approach? Yes, it can work in the short term but tends to fail in the long term. But what else is wrong with it?

What if you're an athlete? What if you're typically a nibbler? What if you have a faster (or slower) than usual metabolism? There is no standard physiology, just like there's no standard person, and so there should be no one-size-fits-all set of recommended portions.

If you're overweight, your current portions (whatever they are) are greater than your body's energy needs. What is the exact portion size your specific physiology needs for its optimal weight set point? There's no way for you to know that yet. But what you can do is move your portions in the direction you need them to go. Remember, this is a dynamic process of eating well. You'll become a healthy eater as you practice these lessons, and control your portions. It doesn't matter how big they are right now. *Not one bit.* But it really does matter that you change them in the right direction day by day.

Hence planning on seconds is an important step. Yes, it gets you to dole out the right amount for your body onto the plate. But that "right" amount will be relative to you—with your personal starting spot for portions—not me, and my arbitrary rules obtained from some new dietary actuarial table.

This initial amount changes as your body adapts to your new behaviors. If you have weight to lose, the portions you put on your plate will drop over time. This is your goal. And it doesn't matter if it takes two days, two weeks, or two months. Some people's bodies will respond right away, and others will adapt over a longer time frame. Each person will proceed at a different rate, just like all of us have different optimal portion sizes.

Be consistent; wait for the change. When you see it, you will know you're making a great stride toward healthy weight loss that will last as long as you need it to.

CHEAT SHEET: Solving Portion Distortion

Remember how your mind and body treat hunger differently? Your body senses your need for food, and your mind drastically amplifies that amount. Your solution is to undershoot your apparent hunger.

- Love your food again—remember what it means to love your food, really.
- Eat small bites so you can taste it more.
- Plan on seconds—put an amount on your plate that you know will be not quite enough, then take your time and enjoy that amount of food.
- Plate size matters—put away large plates forever. Just do it. Eat on medium-size plates and you become a medium-size eater!

The Results You're Looking For

IMMEDIATELY
- You should never be stuffed again.

WITHIN DAYS
- You'll find that your new portions allow you to be satisfied without having to go back for seconds.
- Your estimation of the amount of food your body needs will vary from meal to meal, so don't worry if you don't always get it right.

WITHIN A COUPLE OF WEEKS
- Your mental expectations for the amount of food that seems right will drop as well.

OVER MONTHS

- Your clean-your-plate problem will vanish and you'll be comfortable with walking away from food on your plate.
- You will increase your self-confidence and ability to control portion distortion across a broad spectrum of situations.

HOMEWORK: Eating the Meal

1. Get ready for dinner:
   a. If you live with a family or a group, schedule dinner so you all can eat together. Make the time to take time with them.
   b. If you live alone, treat yourself right. Create a clean, pleasant atmosphere, with candles or background music— whatever you love best.
2. Set the table: Use only medium-size plates.
3. Serve the food: Plan on seconds by underestimating your apparent hunger.
4. During the meal: Take at least twenty minutes to enjoy the meal.
5. After the meal: Relax at the table for about five minutes or more. Then, only if you are not yet full, have a wonderful dessert with your habits of healthy eating.

Don't Eat and Drink at the Same Time

Men who stuff themselves and grow tipsy know neither how to eat nor how to drink.

—JEAN ANTHELME BRILLAT-SAVARIN,
French culinary writer, 1826

Even though eating and drinking are both a part of the meal, you never hear much about the importance of liquids at the table when it comes to weight loss. But as I learned during my time in Lyon, the French have healthy drinking habits that decrease consumption and increase eating pleasure at the same time. These habits come down to some very basic differences between our beliefs about drinking. Let's start with a day in the life of the drinking French.

At the Institute of Cognitive Sciences, we would walk over to eat lunch in the neurological hospital cafeteria. Of all my culture shock moments among the French, my first lunchtime on the job definitely earned a spot in the top ten. My colleagues, of course, thought their cafeteria food to be barely edible (just as we consider ours), but to my American palate, which had been dulled by greasy burgers and fries, the French version of "cafeteria food" easily approached sublime.

Filling the daily lunch tray normally began with a small baguette, followed by the entree and vegetables (Madeira chicken with lightly sautéed green beans with sliced almonds, for example), a small salad of greens or perhaps couscous with olives, a dessert of fruit or fruit tart, and cheese such as Camembert or Brie to round out the meal. Sounds terrible, doesn't it?

After paying and moving to the dining area, a selection of beverages was available ad libitum, including an entire cask of Côtes du Rhône! You could have as much as you wanted. How do I say this more clearly? Free refills of wine . . . in the hospital cafeteria . . . for doctors over lunch.

Now, I grew up in deepest Alabama, where the notion of wine on tap, for doctors, right in the middle of the workday, might tilt the Baptist brain right off the pier, to say the very least. But before we can understand *how* the French consume their liquids, we have to handle a preliminary issue. Why the shock at all? They're not shocked. What was behind my own knee-jerk conclusion that unlimited access to free wine was an insane situation?

This reaction comes from how each of our cultures thinks about this drink. Naturally, the French consume all kinds of nonalcoholic beverages. But wine, of course, is a quintessential part of their dining culture. Parents often give their children a small amount of diluted wine with a meal when they reach a certain age (early teens), and this is seen as a first step into adulthood. It's integral and, as such, is no big deal.

On the other hand, our culture tends to view wine and other alcoholic beverages as "intoxicants." We don't consider them in terms of foods or even drinks, but for their druglike properties. Seen in this way, the point of drinking is to achieve the effect of the drug, subtly (for relaxation, to unwind) or otherwise (to get drunk, blasted, plastered— the synonyms are unfortunately plentiful). We see alcohol, in any form, as a chemical that alters our faculties, and therefore encourages a social danger.

A perfect expression of our social malaise about alcohol is the medical community's reluctance, until lately, to advise a glass of wine to protect the heart. Even before disco, French scientist Serge Renaud's mid-1970s research informed us of wine's heart-protective effects. However, the NIH later objected to his attempt to replicate his Canadian study here in America, citing concerns about "social repercussions." Happy to prescribe an aspirin pill to thin the blood, many physicians remain hampered by an intrinsic fear of wine. This trepidation is quite valid, *but only if we equate drinking alcohol with using a drug.*

And for us, this conservative view makes sense given that our culture equates bigger with better and volume with value. Because we regularly gulp down large quantities of liquids with our meals (more on this later in the step), most of us would agree that it's probably a good thing we don't see wine on tap at the local cafeteria! Thus, our social solution has been to consistently advocate abstinence, while the French rely on responsibility.

But having a glass of wine with a meal each day is an aspect of the French routine that many of us would do well to adopt (assuming we keep it in control). Wine has wonderful health benefits, at a dose of one to two glasses per day, including major reductions in heart disease risk and the recurrence of heart attacks. The massive Copenhagen City Heart Study showed the greatest decrease in mortality, from all causes, to be for wine drinkers versus nondrinkers.

In a 2003 review in *Cardiology Clinics,* it was also pointed out that wine decreases C-reactive protein, which is the most prominent marker for vascular inflammation—*and also associated with obesity.* Today, more than sixty first-rate studies tether a daily glass of wine to health.

That covers the health of your heart, and fits with the way we treat wine as a drug. But what about the notion of having this intoxicant, this depressant, during the workday like the French do? British researchers Lloyd and Rogers at the Institute of Food Research in Reading, U.K., showed in 1997 that "mood and cognitive performance are improved by a small amount of alcohol given with a lunchtime meal." In fact, their research demonstrated that the most productive thing employees could do for their afternoon productivity would be to have a beer or glass of wine over the noontime meal.

No kidding. A small amount of alcohol improved the attentiveness of employees better than a high level of alcohol, and even more than having none at all!

All this already makes sense to the French, who consider wine in the same way as food. Very simply, it attends the meal. Its potentially intoxicating properties are lost on no one, of course, but intoxication is not the point. One drinks wine for its pleasing complement to the palate and plate.

Seen in this light, a glass of Bordeaux over lunch is as acceptable as it is obvious. By the way, remember the free, all-you-can-drink wine cask? I never saw anyone sloppy, nor anyone beating a path back for multiple trips to the cask (and I had my Alabama eyes peeled).

The key to enjoyment and good health is moderation—for all your drinks as well as your food. But here's the kicker—when it comes to effortless weight loss, wine's benefit is about more than just the alcohol or heart-healthy polyphenols. It's about volume control at all levels of consumption. *Wine naturally encourages moderation during mealtimes because you have to sip it.* And learning to control the quantity of your drinks turns out to be a solution to control the size of your food portions as well. The case in point is a fact typical of the drinking American—the "toilet bowl effect."

Super Big Gulping: The Toilet Bowl Effect

I get calls from all over. One particular call came from a woman in Kansas who had read *The Fat Fallacy* and had a few questions. We chatted for a while about food and health and weight. She eventually noted that she grew up in Dothan, Alabama, just like I did. Getting a phone call out of the blue from someone who grew up in my hometown was a little like seeing a falling star in a leap year. Her maiden name was Carpenter. "I didn't know any Carpenters, except my old baseball coach, the chiropractor with about six kids," I said.

"He was my father!" she exclaimed. After catching up on mutual acquaintances, she mentioned an interesting quirk about how her father ate: Dr. Carpenter didn't like them to have anything to drink at the table with the meal.

Okay, I thought. "Why not?"

She went on to explain that it was precisely because of the "toilet bowl effect." Her father hated to see people get their mouths so full of food that they needed a tumbler of water just to flush it all back, and so they were allowed a beverage before or after a meal, but not during. Once she explained it, this made so much sense to me. The simple rules for drinks should be the same as those for food. Don't gulp your drink, don't gulp your food.

In fact, remember the rule of thumb from Step 4? The analogous rule for drinks is to sip your drink. Okay, I hear your questions already . . . and no, there's no exact measurement that's the perfect sip volume.

Remember that this French Don't Diet Plan you've now begun retrains your healthy behaviors. Where the first rule is to eat small, that applies just as well to the huge drink sizes we face every day. Just sit down to eat in any restaurant, and they'll bring you an enormous glass of whatever you want. Step inside a convenience store and you can walk out with practically a drum full of any beverage for just forty-nine cents. Even at home, we pour drinks into large glasses when we eat. The volume of liquid we consume is too large and unfortunately flies under the radar of our weight and health strategies: We never even consider this an important issue!

But let's say you're avoiding high-calorie beverages and drink only water. Surely there can't be any problem with downing lots of water every day—it has no calories, right? That's true, but remember the French approach: It's not just *what* you consume; *how* you consume it matters every bit as much. The habit of eating and drinking large quantities of anything, even water, can affect your weight and health.

Water is a perfect example of a drink that's indisputably good for you, but in excess it can cause trouble. For example, take professional competitive eater Eric "Badlands" Booker. Eric is one of these people who goes from town to town to show how many hot dogs or pizzas or oysters he can ingest in a certain amount of time. It's great theater, like professional wrestling or the sword swallower at the circus, but don't try this at home.

Meal Drinks

Some drinks, such as tea, coffee, and wine, really lend themselves to sipping. Beer, water, milk, and juice can be overconsumed by gulping, so you have to practice your healthy habits with these.

Like others of his ilk, he trains by expanding his stomach capacity. Do you know how they do this? Not by eating, but by drinking. Each day for two or three days before "meets," he drinks a gallon of water.

Professional eater "Crazy Legs" Conti goes even further. In a recent interview, he stated that he would drink a gallon of water in under two minutes and even swallow ice cubes to stretch his esophagus.

Here's the problem: When you flush your meals down with a lot of liquid, you can inadvertently expand your capacity for eating in greater volumes. Thus, consuming more liquid actually primes our bodies to take in higher quantities of food over the long term.

Of the incredible number of factors that cause weight problems (besides just calories in, calories out), the toilet bowl effect is perhaps the most overlooked. But if you are serious about controlling consumption, and thereby calories, and thereby weight, you've got to train in the habits of healthy drinking as well.

Ending the Toilet Bowl Effect

You're going to move in the opposite direction from the extremes of eating and the extremes of drinking. Instead of training your body to increase your eating capacity, you're going to further decrease it *without deprivation*. In this step, you'll form the new drinking habits that free your body up for natural weight loss.

Thirst and the Mind-Body Connection

"[Thirst] is regulated by the central nervous system and arises from neural and chemical signals from the periphery interacting in the brain to stimulate a drive to drink. . . . Osmotic and hormonal stimuli from the circulation are detected by neurons in this region and how that information is integrated with other neural signals to generate thirst" (McKinley, 2004).

SCIENCE-TO-ENGLISH TRANSLATION

True bodily thirst signals get transported to the brain. Then they're "interpreted" before you feel the thirst.

But before we can conquer the toilet bowl effect, we've got to understand what's going on here. Face it, we eat when we're not hungry and drink when we're not thirsty. Consumption is driven by something else—visual cues, emotional baggage, who knows. It could be anything. The point is that a healthy relationship with food and drink requires us to relearn to recognize the natural sensations of the body.

Just as your body's hunger gets amplified by your mind (you feel like you "could eat a horse," but it's just not true) your sensations for thirst are altered as well. For example, the subjects in a 2004 study published in *Physiological Behavior* were tested during a normal workday. Here's the question investigated by the scientists: "Is thirst just a product of dehydration?"

The answer is no. Blood samples were taken every hour from healthy young men who also rated how thirsty they were. The researchers found that the perception of thirst came even when the body was not "thirsty." Specifically, subjects didn't have the blood markers for low hydration and yet (especially when eating) something else had generated the apparent thirst. *"The results indicate that during free access to water humans become thirsty and drink before body fluid deficits develop."*

More studies show that, when you drink very quickly, your sensation of "quenching your thirst" results from filling up your belly with liquid, not from changing the hydration level of your bodily fluids. This leads to mixed signals when drinking too much too fast.

Sound familiar?

The point is not that you shouldn't drink water, but to understand that your signals for drinking are like those for hunger, and are filtered when they go from body to mind. The link between these pairs, just like the link between high-quality and low-quantity eating, keeps returning over and over in the French approach, in what they eat, how they eat, and even how they drink. Before you can get to this point though, we have to overcome some of our most ingrained biases and myths. These coach us to consume more and, when we do, to train our bodies to expect more over the long term.

⚜ PEOPLE ON THE PATH

Dear Dr. Clower,

I do wish I had learned about this way of eating sooner. You see, I have just been diagnosed with stage 1 breast cancer and am scheduled for surgery at the beginning of February. I strongly believe that my years of low-fat/no-fat eating robbed my body of the protective nutrients it needed to fight off cancer. In addition, this same mentality convinced me that prepackaged food laden with chemicals was the healthy choice for weight control, the same chemicals that may have also contributed to my cancer.

Over the years, I've lost twenty-five pounds, fifty pounds, fifty pounds, and this last time twenty pounds. I was desperate for a plan that would help me keep the weight off. (Sound familiar?)

Reading your work was like having a locked door suddenly unlock and free me from the trap I seemed to live in. Since April, I have kept the weight off (in fact, I lost an additional five to six pounds) while enjoying my food more but eating less. I no longer fear food or look at it like it's something I must grudgingly endure. I feel confident for the first time ever since losing weight that I can keep it off.

I am thrilled to be a convert to a new lifestyle that allows me to enjoy food without the neurotic obsession that permeates our fat-phobic society. I have been living this lifestyle since last April, and I can tell you that it works for me.

My thanks to you, Dr. Clower!

—*Dianna R.*

The Myth of Eight Glasses of Water per Day

But wait, you say. Aren't you *supposed* to drink at least eight glasses of water every day? Shouldn't you carry around a quart of water with you wherever you go, clipped to your belt so you can down a bit more at every occasion . . . including your meals? You have to stay hydrated, right?

The kernel of this widely reported fallacy is actually quite true. Dehydration is a covert source of many health problems and you do need water to stay healthy. Moreover, we lose water daily through our breath, sweat, and when we go to the bathroom. We can offset that loss and stay hydrated only through oral intake.

Everyone agrees up to this point. But the notion of "eight glasses" has been taken to an extreme that science has since put the brakes on. For example, Dr. Heinz Valtin of Dartmouth Medical School performed an exhaustive review of all work done on the subject. Here's what he found: "Despite the seemingly ubiquitous admonition to 'drink at least eight 8-oz glasses of water a day' (with an accompanying reminder that beverages containing caffeine and alcohol do not count), rigorous proof for this counsel appears to be lacking."

This is the kind of conservative language you find in a peer-reviewed science paper. Another way to say it is that this advice has all been a big fat myth. After all, the health media is not just telling you to drink water, but that you must drink *at least* eight eight-ounce glasses of water every day! So people carry quart-sized bottles and tank up on their daily allotment like a Labrador getting ready for a long walk.

Dr. Valtin's results state a little more emphatically later on that "surveys of food and fluid intake on thousands of adults of both genders, analyses of which have been published in peer-reviewed journals, strongly suggest that such large amounts are not needed."

His results square exactly with the behavior of the French, who drink water with their meals in small glasses, not quart bottles.

So the truth is somewhere in the middle. You do need water. You just don't need to drown in it to be healthy. Remember that a tomato is 90 percent water, as are most denizens of a common tossed salad. Unless you're eating nothing but dry, powdered food, you're likely getting water from your meal as well. And you take in the most water when you eat foods such as fruits and veggies.

Another important point concerns the diuretic effect of drinks containing alcohol and caffeine. Drinks such as tea, beer, and coffee contain water, obviously, but they also pull water out of your body. This can be confusing—what is the balance? Are they water-positive or water-negative? The answer is that you actually gain more water than you lose, so you don't need to drink extra water to make up for their effects.

The Science of the Water Myth

Drs. Grandjean and colleagues compared equal volumes of many kinds of drinks on the state of hydration: changes in body weight and standard urinary and plasma variables. The drinks included water, caffeinated and noncaffeinated, caloric and noncaloric beverages. There were no significant effects on any measure of hydration. The authors concluded that *"advising people to disregard caffeinated beverages as part of the daily fluid intake is not substantiated by the results"* (Grandjean, 2000).

It's important to point out that if you're among those who are very active or are out in the hot sun all day, you'll lose a lot more water to sweat, and so must drink more fluids to compensate. On a recent trip to Vail, Colorado, I was advised to drink a little water because it's very easy to become dehydrated in the thin air. Additional water is also very necessary for those who are ill. But if you're in the broad middle of the cubicle worker population who are basically healthy, sedentary, and not too sweaty, you can safely drink less than we've been told.

⚜ *Problem: How do you find the healthy middle ground with your drinks? And how can your drinking habits positively influence your eating habits and, ultimately, your weight?*

Solution 1: Don't eat and drink at the same time.

The French definitely drink water or wine or both with their meals, so what about the idea of not having anything to drink with your meal? Frankly, it sounded as weird to me as self-serve refills on wine for doctors over lunch so, hey, I decided to give it a shot. And to my surprise, I found this technique to be a perfect training tool for healthy eating habits—which are directly affected by your drinking habits.

Try this as your homework this week: eat your dinner without a drink. I know it seems strange at first, but just try it. You'll find that you've got enough saliva in your mouth naturally, and your food has enough moisture, that you don't actually need a drink at all. Eat small and you can swallow without incident, without having to flush it down your throat.

If you have trouble swallowing, your bite was too big. That's how you know.

Solution 2: Sip your drinks.

Once you've eliminated drinks at meals for a day or two, add them back and practice sipping. At that point, your drink becomes something you include because you love the taste or how it goes with the food. That's exactly how you follow the French habits of eating at the table. In other words, you'll choose your drink because you love the way it tastes or complements the meal, not because you need assistance swallowing.

From now on, taste your drink. Sip, never gulp! Never fill your mouth full of anything, including the liquid you drink. This must become ingrained, so practice the behavioral habit. Each time you pick up your drink, or put straw to lips, sip from it. Whenever you do this, you train your body to expect less volume in the long term.

Solution 3: Try smaller drink sizes.

You will find it easier to sip when the volume in front of you is small. Remember, your body is probably half as thirsty as your brain says you are. So when you buy a drink, always get a small one, not the medium size that's huge by traditional standards, and certainly not the fifty-five-gallon drum with the straw in it! To follow this French lifestyle approach, it's important to buy small, drink small, and make that amount last over a longer time.

Likewise, it doesn't matter how extra-tired you think you are, you don't need the extra-large coffee. You don't need to drink that much fluid, nor do you need that much caffeine—even if you think you do. The grande coffee from Starbucks has an eye-popping 550 milligrams of caffeine in it! And just like your caffeine tolerance goes up, drinking that much coffee just trains your body to expect that amount every time.

By the way, the syrupy milkshakes disguised as coffee? With the caramel or fudge or other syrup in them? Please don't buy these. You might as well eat Karo syrup by the spoon. And don't think you can just order this calorie explosion with low-fat or skim milk in it, because that won't counteract the high-fructose corn syrup and make it all healthy again. This is no different than downing a diet soda with a bar of taffy and thinking that they cancel each other out somewhere in your lower gastric world!

Don't Forget, Don't Diet

Because for years our standard fad diets have overlooked the big picture, we have missed a critical factor contributing to our weight and health problems—not just food, but drinks as well.

Relearning "how to drink" is a great example of how basic healthy principles can benefit you in many ways. First, relearning to drink small by sipping frees you from excess fluid consumption. Next, this training reinforces your habits of eating small as well, so the amount of food and drink your body asks for will drop over time.

By this method, you can avoid the toilet bowl effect. Even better is the change you'll find in your appreciation of food. When your drink is merely functional—used to fire hose your lunch down—it drowns out the flavor of the food. You can't enjoy it and you're certainly not drinking for taste or pleasure. You're solving a problem created by your eating habits.

All these small factors add up to producing lower weight for life. And, because you're learning new habits, they continue to work for you even after you forget about them.

CHEAT SHEET: How to Drink

This lifestyle approach to weight control relies on some very intuitive principles: Eat well. Love what you consume. Take your time. Overconsumption (of anything) is bad for you. Moderation will save your life. And all that goes for your drinks as well.

- Water is good, but most healthy people don't need "at least eight eight-ounce glasses" each day.
- Always sip your drink, whether water, wine, tea, juice, or beer.
- Practice not eating and drinking at the same time.
- Swallow your food before you take a drink. That way, you'll never use your drink to wash back your food.
- Always buy the small drink size. Take your time and enjoy what you have.

The Results You're Looking For

IMMEDIATELY
- You will reinforce your habits of eating small.
- You will enjoy your food more.
- You will find it easier to eat small when you're drinking small as well.

WITHIN A WEEK

- You will become aware that you never needed more than a small drink anyway.
- You will not need to carry a bottle of water around with you.

HOMEWORK: DRINKING

1. Practice eating at the table without a drink, to overcome the toilet bowl effect.
2. You also use this exercise as your practice for eating small. If you have trouble swallowing, your bite was too big.
3. Practice your habits of healthy drinking:

    a. Only sip, never gulp.

    b. If there's food in your mouth, set your drink down.
4. Buy only small-size drinks.

Eat All You Want
(You'll Just Want Less)

Whenever I'm asked about how often we should eat during the day, I remember a particular experience I had visiting the Mediterranean coast. On an impulse to go south and smell the Provence sea air, Dottie, the kids, and I hopped in the car for a long weekend trip to the little coastal village of Sète, about three hours from Lyon. It was a brilliant blue day, and we were determined to get to Sète as quickly as possible to make the most of our mini-vacation. By the time we arrived, we had worked up a good solid hunger since we hadn't bothered to stop for lunch. So off we went to find a restaurant at three in the afternoon.

At the very first one, we noticed a waiter standing out on the patio overlooking a cyan sea that almost matched the cloudless sky. I was ready for a long communion with that view. We practically skipped up, startling him with our puppy-like eagerness to sit down for lunch.

"*Non, non,*" he said with the patience of a kindergarten teacher accustomed to explaining the most basic realities of life. He looked at his watch before slowly returning his gaze to us. "*C'est finis.* Lunch is over. It's three o'clock."

Our embarrassing lesson? The French eat at mealtimes and mealtimes are when they eat.

This, of course, is so contrary to our normal habits of chronic consumption and noshing all through the day. Incessant eating has even turned into health advice, with the most recent faddish theory telling you to go ahead and snack all the time—every three hours. "You should eat six or more meals per day," experts have said. (The problem is, we're doing this already!)

It reminds me of Eisenhower's response when asked how to be a good parent. "Oh, that's easy," quipped Ike. "You just find out what your kids want, then advise them to go do that."

The theory of eating all day long is interesting in an academic sense: You have to keep your insulin levels up so you don't get hungry so you don't have to eat all the time (say, every three hours). But what culture grazes all day long except Americans (whose obesity rate is greater than 30 percent)? The Japanese (whose obesity rate is 5 percent), Italians (whose obesity rate is 12 percent), and French (whose obesity rate is 12 percent) don't consume their way through the morning and afternoon. In fact, the French eat only two and a half meals per day.

If you want to eat like thin, healthy people, eat for pleasure, and get their results, you have to do what they do: Eat only during meal times.

Science of the French Lifestyle

In a recent issue of *Obesity Surgery*, "grazing" was classified as a high-risk behavior. And it indicated a disturbed eating pattern similar to bingeing in patients who have undergone gastric bypass. In fact, patients often just substituted bingeing for grazing *(Saunders, 2004).*

When I worked in Lyon, the break room at our research building had no snack machine. There was a refrigerator with people's lunches and some coffee in it. But there were no banks of vending machine options for the candies and chips we've become used to. (There *were* plenty of people at the coffee machine, but they just don't snack like we do.)

So how do you stop snacking without being hungry all day long?

How do you get from where you are now to where you want to be, painlessly? The answer comes right back to the intuitive eating habits the French have been enjoying for the past few centuries. And perhaps the most decadent and delicious part of their meal is the "ender," the final mouthwatering morsel that also helps end the between-meal cravings that drive total consumption through the roof.

The Best Kept Secret of the French Approach: "The Ender"

To be able to eat all you want (but just want less) is your goal. And the easiest, most sumptuous strategy for getting there is to punctuate the pleasure of the meal with a little something extra—a rich delicious portion—after you've finished the main part of your meal.

How do you define the ender? Think of it as the exclamation mark of eating enjoyment. I'm certain this fantastic French habit didn't become a part of their eating routine to control snacking. But this is exactly the effect it has. When practiced right, the physiological consequence is that you *will no longer feel hungry between meals.* This, of course, makes you consume fewer calories, which in turn makes you lose more weight. And it's the best kept secret of the entire French approach.

Here's what you do: After you've finished your lunch or dinner, wait ten minutes. If you can somehow manage to sit and relax for the eon of ten whole minutes, do that—it's good for your digestion! If you have ants in your pants and have to *do something* all the time, put away the food, the dishes, and then sit back down for your ender. But the preferred method is definitely to sit and enjoy the last of your wine and the company you keep.

After the ten minutes have passed, have your ender. The ender is a calorie-dense bit of oral bliss, so keep the amount under control. Your instructions are to enjoy it, absolutely guilt-free.

I'm told so often by our PATH participants that they love the ender because it's their signal that the meal is over. After you've had it, you'll find that you don't want any more food until dinner (or tomorrow's breakfast) because you've reached the end of the meal. Think of it as a stop sign and you can create the correct mental association.

Wonderful example enders include cheeses, rich chocolates, and nuts. Liquid enders include coffee and tea. I'll spend a little time talking about each of these.

Cheeses

Almost any cheese is rich enough to satisfy as an ender, so just choose your favorite. Brie, Camembert, or any variety that has no hydrogenated oil or the words *food product* on the label are wonderful. If you've never tried these before, I recommend starting out with a basic Brie. (You don't have to eat the rind, just trim it off if you like.) From there, you can branch off to any variety at all—although blue cheese can be a little strong for an ender, especially if you're planning on coming within three feet of someone anytime soon.

Shop for cheese enders in specialty stores that feature a wide variety of them or in supermarkets that have their own cheese sections, where you'll find the best ones.

As you eat the cheese, try not to use your teeth on the softer varieties and only nibble on the harder ones. Just work it over in your mouth so you can make the taste last as long as possible. This lets you enjoy the rich flavor, while keeping the amount low enough to make sure it stays healthy for you.

DO END WITH: Any rich delicious cheese that you like.

DON'T END WITH: Cheese product, cheese food, Cheez Whiz, or plastic-wrapped American singles.

HOW MUCH: Remember the rule of thumb, and have no more than two thumbs' worth, or a piece the size of four dice.

Chocolates

The botanical name for chocolate translates as "food of the gods." Who is really surprised by this? Chocolate makes an excellent ender—and is a favorite of the French. The key is not to settle for bulk chocolate, which can contain fillers, partially hydrogenated oils, and corn syrups. Remember, you avoid high-quantity eating when you choose high-quality foods. So get the most natural chocolate you can find—it's much better for you.

Next, keep in mind that the part of the chocolate that's good for you is the cocoa itself, and the part that's bad is the fake oils and sugar. So choose a dark, natural chocolate (the darker the better). Most healthy food stores such as Whole Foods or Trader Joes will carry delicious dark chocolates from places like France and Belgium, but if your town doesn't have a store with good varieties, you can also order any variety on the planet, online, from places such as Chocosphere (www.chocosphere.com).

When you eat your chocolate, never chew it. Chocolate melts in your mouth very slowly, which means that even a very small amount will gradually and steadily give off its flavor, leaving you with chocolate, and chocolate, and more chocolate. And after all that delicious flavor, all you will have had is one very small piece.

DO END WITH: Dark chocolate, preferably French or Belgian.

DON'T END WITH: White chocolate, light milk chocolate, anything other than solid chocolate (no candy bars, wafers, or chocolate-coated candies), or anything that contains hydrogenated oil or high-fructose corn syrup.

HOW MUCH: Two thumb-size squares.

Nuts

Eating nuts as an ender is not a French tradition, but it is an innovation that works very well. Make sure the nuts you choose are unsalted (the salty ones make you crave more). Wonderful candidates include Brazil nuts, cashews, walnuts, and almonds. By the way, in addition to helping you stave off between-meal snacking, their oils are very good for your heart.

I spoke with one woman on the phone who really wanted to make the ender work for her, and called me to troubleshoot why it wasn't working. Her appetite was not settling down between meals and (because she was still grazing through the day) her weight just wasn't coming off. When I asked what she was having as her ender, she simply informed me that she was doing exactly as I recommended and was having a few nuts.

"Nuts. What kind?" I asked.

"Oh, those honey-roasted Boston baked beans. They're wonderful."

So we had to have a conversation about sugar and I pointed out that, even if you're having healthy foods, if you're drowning them in sugar and preservatives and Red No. 40 dye, you're not going to make much progress! Many food products seem healthy, but you have to make sure they really are by reading the labels.

DO END WITH: The nuts you enjoy the best, as long as they are unsalted.

DON'T END WITH: Candy bars with nuts or sweetened honey-roasted varieties.

HOW MUCH: No more than the size of your palm (so you might have eight almonds, but only five Brazil nuts, for example).

Ender Drinks

A little coffee or tea serves as a wonderful ender. Especially when you've just had dessert—you don't need both an ender and a dessert when you're trying to shed pounds. Just like the rule for food enders, liquid enders can be overdone when you order, so never get the large size and never get versions with any added sugar.

Coffee, at a level of one to three small cups per day, also acts as a wonderful appetite suppressant. In addition to its healthy antioxidants, it also seems to stabilize your insulin levels. This, in fact, may help explain just how it stops between-meal cravings.

Why the Ender Works

Why does this delicious French habit work? Physiologically, the natural fiber and oils of the ender accomplish two important things for your digestion. First, they slow the rate that your stomach empties into your small intestine (where your food will be absorbed into your blood-stream). Slowing this rate down stabilizes your insulin levels because the food is absorbed more gradually. The oils also trigger hormonal satiety signals, such as cholecystokinin, which go to your brain and say, "I'm satisfied, you can stop eating now."

That's how the ender conquers between-meal cravings on three fronts: It becomes your mental association for the meal's end, helps stabilize blood sugar, and sends the message of satisfaction to your brain. In fact, not only is the ender one reason the French approach leaves people satisfied without having to eat all the time, we have seen this habit help alleviate the symptoms of hypoglycemia for our clients on the PATH Healthy Eating Curriculum.

But don't forget that you can mess this up by having too much of a good thing. In other words, the wonderful satiety effect of your rich ender can decrease *if you have too much of it*. When that happens, you will consistently have to eat more to get the same hunger-relieving ef-fect. Don't go down that path; keep your ender small to keep it healthy and effective.

Managing Between-Meal Hunger Blips

The ender becomes your bridge from one meal to the next, freeing you from nagging hunger. But even with the ender, you may still face between-meal cravings from time to time (especially in the first few weeks). You can easily manage these interim cravings, but you have to understand what they actually are because so many people misinter-pret these sensations.

We've already talked about how much our mind overestimates true hunger and thirst. The same thing happens with your between-meal pangs. Here's what you need to remember: Hunger comes in little waves. Its first sensations are small and last just a couple of minutes be-fore they go away. And when they're gone, you're not hungry anymore.

These are authentic hunger feelings. But when you're in the middle of a hunger blip, you normally don't realize that it's just passing through and lasts only a few minutes. All you know is the feeling of urgency, with delusions of spending the next few hours in a state of stomach-grinding famine. And the gnawing feeling prevents you from getting any work done, because you can't get thoughts of the snack machine out of your head. In this little mental microcosm, your desk items start looking tasty!

Extrapolation is the problem here. You think that, because you've just become this hungry, you'll get even hungrier over the next three hours before the meal. But the hunger blip lasts only a couple of minutes before you're freed from having to launch yourself into the break room fridge. It's just a blip.

It's truly amazing when you get to the other side of this little hunger snag and realize that it's gone. Where did it go? It makes you wonder if it was ever real at all. Of course the feeling was real—you felt it. But how could you be that annoyingly hungry one minute and then "not hungry at all" the next? This tells you, loud and clear, that your hunger feelings are *interpretations* of your body's needs—not your body's needs. It's an apparition that you can let go.

Don't leap at the ghosts of hunger. Wait them out and let them pass.

Simple Solutions for Getting over Hunger Blips

- Did you quit smoking by going cold turkey? If you're this kind of all-or-nothing person with strong self-discipline, just be patient and wait out the little hunger pang. After all, you know it's going away in a few minutes anyway. So distract yourself with your job or a conversation or a walk outside until you've bumped over the blip and it's gone. This is the best-case scenario.

- Another strategy, for the orally fixated, is to have a small cup of water. Health professionals say that sometimes thirst can seem like hunger, and you should drink some water when you feel hungry. Essentially, it takes three or four minutes for you to get up, get the water, and sip it. In that three to four minutes, the blip is gone anyway! It works, but may not have anything to do your thirst seeming like hunger. More likely, you're just giving your blip a chance to fade away on its own.

- At the other extreme, if you're melting down like the witch in *The Wizard of Oz*, "Aahh, what a world, what a world," and you can't stand it anymore, by all means have a snack. Any of the enders make wonderful snacks, but you must look at this as something to get you over the blip and through the afternoon. Do not eat to fill up. After you've had a little something, notice when your cravings go away again.

Starting today, experiment with your between-meal blip. Everyone's hunger profile will be different, so find out what yours is like. Time how long it lasts, and write down what you do that pulls you through it.

When you understand your cravings better, the first thing you'll likely notice is that sugary foods at the meal inflame your between-meal blip—making it larger and longer. Sugar stimulates an insulin surge, which whisks the energy reserves out of your blood and into your muscles and organs where (it thinks) you need it. After that happens, you feel like you're low on energy again.

On the other hand, meals with natural fiber, protein, or fat guard against between-meal hunger. So when you have breakfast, for example, have something natural: apples are better than apple juice because the sugar is accompanied by fiber; normal milk is better than skim because it's accompanied by a higher level of fat; whole-grain breads are better than sugary white bread . . . you get the picture.

❖ PEOPLE ON THE PATH

Dear Dr. Clower,

I think I began doing sit-ups and sleeping with Teen magazine at about nine years old. That's when it began. I proceeded to feel a little too heavy, specifically in my belly, for the next eighteen years or so. I tried hating myself, loving myself, starving myself, eating whatever I wanted, eating vegan, praying, head-banging . . . but to no avail.

So, when I happened to find out about this approach, something clicked. I didn't know it right away, but life was sailing toward the land of quite fabulous.

I had slaved my way through South Beach and other such atrocities before I came to. I think it was during a downpour on a spring evening when I woke up: Life is not about dietary control. There is a way to live passionately and presently, whether it's about food, work, men, or bills. I kid, but it's true: at least on the topic of food. . . . The war is over.

The result? Size 6 or 8 from a 12 or 14. Yay! No more panic attacks over bloating! No more inner commentary! And for the first time since I was nine years old, a natural connection with food, my body, and unadulterated joy.

Take care,
Jennifer C.

P.S. My mother has started as well, and I don't think she's looked so fabulous since I was very young. It's so much fun to have a partner in my lifestyle weight loss!

Why Snacking Makes You Want to Eat Even More: The Appetite Thermometer

The principle bears repeating. You respond to your body's cravings by eating. But your body's cravings are created by your eating behaviors. It's a circle.

Every step we've taken so far shows how to retrain these behaviors to serve you—for your portions, drinks, and even your between-meal cravings. Now we're going to give you the tools to track this change and push your overall hunger level lower with the appetite thermometer, or appestat. This idea has been around for at least fifty years (the first paper I've found on it dates back to 1952, and discusses the early ideas about the brain mechanisms of appetite regulation).

You don't have to get caught up in too many details to understand how this works. Just remember that the appestat is simply all the body chemicals that get released after you eat, which sum up in your brain to create feelings of hunger and fullness.

You can think about your body's appetite thermometer just like the thermostat you have in your home that controls temperature. When the air cools, the heater comes on until the temperature reaches the set level and then it cuts off. The same thing happens in your body. When your energy gets low, your hunger mechanisms kick in to make you eat until you pass the thermometer threshold. If your appetite thermometer is set high, you'll be hungry for a lot of food. If it's low, you're one of those people who eats like a bird.

And, just like when your mother-in-law comes over and cranks the thermostat *way* up, your body has its own nefarious influences that can change yours (I'm sure I didn't mean to associate *nefarious* with *mother-in-law*, I'm sure I meant *wonderful*). Although your mother-in-law may control your home thermometer, you get to regulate your personal appetite mechanism. In fact, the ability to dial it up or down empowers most people who live this lifestyle. Changing your level of hunger is the long-term lifestyle solution for ultimate portion control.

Turn down the appestat so your body will ask for less food. When you do this, you can eat all you want. You just want less. *That's the secret that explains this part of the French paradox.*

Making the Measurement

At least for this week, keep a diary. There are only two measurements you'll need to take: your eating volume, and the number of times you eat during the day. In other words, it's the *volume* your body needs over *time*. If you reduce the amount you eat or increase the time between meals, you effectively dial down your body's appetite thermometer. For you math-heads, here's an equation to describe it:

Volume (portions) / Time between eating (minutes) × 100

(We just multiply by 100 to make it a convenient number to read.)

TIME BETWEEN ONE MEAL AND THE NEXT: This is easy—just add up the minutes. Start with breakfast and note how much time passes between breakfast and the next time you eat—whether it's lunch or a between-meal snack. Did you make it from breakfast, ending at nine A.M., to lunch, starting at one P.M.? That's four hours, or 240 minutes, without hunger. Did you have to have a snack between the two meals around eleven A.M.? Simple. In that case, you'd write down 120 minutes (2 hours) without being hungry.

Do the same between lunch and dinner. If you finish lunch at one, and then don't eat until dinner at five, that's four hours—240 minutes. If you have to snack at three, that's two hours, or 120 minutes.

Now you just add up the two times: 240 minutes from breakfast to lunch plus 240 minutes from lunch to dinner. That's 480 minutes total.

FOOD VOLUME IS JUST AS EASY: Approximate and add up the volume of food you eat in a day. Don't worry, you don't have to calculate grams or carry around a scale or anything silly like that. Just estimate the portions on your plate by using a measurement, such as the size of a deck of cards or your fist as one portion, as listed in our portions chart in Step 5 as a guide.

For example, if you have an egg for breakfast, that's one portion. If you also had a bowl of oatmeal (about two-thirds full), that's one portion. Add one piece of toast with butter, that's three portions at breakfast.

Do the same with lunch. If you have a serving of meat, a veggie, and a starch, that's three portions. Add a dessert and you've had four portions for lunch. Get the idea? Then if you have four of these portions for dinner, you've had a total of eleven (three at breakfast, four at lunch, and four at dinner). That's all. The math's pretty simple, too.

Example: Kim's Appestat Reading

Kim ate at mealtimes and didn't snack.

Volume in portions:

2 (breakfast) + 4 (lunch) + 4 (dinner) = 10 portions

Time between meals in minutes:

240 (4 hours from breakfast to lunch) + 240 (4 hours from lunch to dinner) = 480 minutes

Appestat reading:

(10 portions / 480 minutes) × 100 = 2.1

Example: David's Appestat Reading

David snacked on a doughnut between breakfast and lunch, but then didn't eat until dinner. He had dessert.

Volume in portions:

2 (breakfast) + 1 (snack) + 3 (lunch) + 4 (dinner) + 1 (dessert) = 11 portions

Time between meals:

120 (2 hours from breakfast to snack) + 240 (4 hours from lunch to dinner) = 360 minutes

Appestat reading:

(11 portions / 120 minutes) × 100 = 3.1

When you snack between meals, your appestat goes higher. I guess a better way of saying this is, when your appestat is higher, you snack between meals. In these two examples alone it went up from 2.1 to 3.1.

Let's review this for the mathematically disinclined. As you can see, all we're doing is adding up the amount you eat through the day. That's your total intake. We compare this to how often you have to eat. Thus, it's your body's food volume over time. And this feeding rate amounts to what your body is asking for—your basic appetite threshold.

Don't Be Exact, Just Be Consistent

Everyone who's ever been on a diet panics when I tell them to estimate portions. Is the mashed potato portion about the size of a deck of cards, or a shade larger, or maybe it's a regulation deck of cards, or, or . . . I was overseas once, and they have cards that are longer and thinner . . . ?

Don't worry—you don't need to sweat the details. However you estimate portions is fine, as long as you consistently use the same estimations each time. The appetite thermometer is just helping you track the changes and push the bar lower.

Interpret the Appestat Reading

The reason that you don't have to be an accountant with your portions is because your appetite thermometer reading is a relative number. *It has meaning only when you see how it changes, week by week.*

I'm not going to tell you how many portions you should have. Just have the amount you're hungry for, and then watch that amount change over time as you dial down your appestat. I don't have to dictate your portions as they do on standard diets, because your current hunger level (or appestat setting) is not important whatsoever right now. What is important is that you move the setting in the correct direction—down, not up! So you can be at peace with where you are right now, and move your body's cravings in the direction you want them to go.

Remember, this is about the process of putting your body in training to relearn healthy eating habits for life. As with anything you would train for, you cannot start at the end, and the training process takes time.

So when you add up your appestat reading, start from a week's average value. Don't worry when your daily readings fluctuate dramatically. These micro changes don't matter as much as the larger changes that happen from week to week.

Dial Down Your Cravings

Identify key areas that push your appetite lower. These include the number of portions at a sitting and the tendency to snack between meals. Everyone is different, but here are some suggested portion values you will work your way toward: breakfast, 2 portions; lunch, 3 portions; dinner, 4 portions; snacks, 0.

WHAT DIALS DOWN YOUR APPETITE THERMOMETER?

Every time you eat small.

Every time you stop eating when you are satisfied.

Every time you push the portion bar lower.

Every time you go between meals without snacking.

Every time your meal includes food with natural levels of fiber, fat, and protein.

Every time you take your time and enjoy your meal.

Every time you solve the clean-your-plate problem.

WHAT TURNS YOUR APPETITE THERMOMETER UP?

Every time you rush through a meal.

Every time you eat sugary foods.

Every time you eat when you're stressed.

Every time you graze through the afternoon.

Every time you eat so much that you feel stuffed after a meal.

Own Your Own Health

In the last three steps, we talked about how to solve portion distortion so your eating habits control eating volume for you. And now with the lessons learned in this step, you can master chronic overeating as well. Put these together and you have a clear message of hope. No longer will you diet over and over only to regain weight. You really can change what your body asks for so it asks for less and leaves you healthier in the process.

But how do you get from where you are now to where you want to be? How do you make the transition from the engrained habits that frustrate your attempts at weight loss, and replace them with the success of the French approach? It starts by realizing what you can change, what you can't, and what you have to be at peace with.

To Change Your Body, Change Your Mind

Some things must be accepted. Some things can be changed. Meditation can slow autonomic functions such as heart rate, or even blood pressure. Korean (Hae-Nyo) and Japanese (Ama) sponge and pearl divers have actually changed their physiology so they can hold their breath an incredible two minutes. Of course, there are limits to what biological knobs and buttons you can push and pull in your own body, but many more aspects are malleable than you think.

It takes just a minute to realize what this means. Our body may limit us, but we can push the envelope of those boundaries if we choose. Our urges may drive us to behave in unhealthy ways, but our behavior sculpts those urges.

For example:

Long-distance runners have great lung capacity, so they can run a
    long way.
    But they got that capacity *because they run.*
Brilliant singers have angelic voices, so they can sing.
    But they got those voices *because they sing.*
People crave sweets because they have sweet tooths.
    But they got those sweet tooths *because they eat sweets.*

You get the picture. You can nudge your own desires in a positive or negative direction, very easily grow sweet cravings by consistently eating oversugared foods, or create a huge appetite by eating tons of food.

But here's the good news. If you find yourself within this pit of self-inflicted health problems, you can still get out of it through your own efforts. And don't worry if it takes a while. You didn't slide into this hole overnight; so don't expect to climb out with one magic pill, fat-be-gone ring, or fad diet. It's not going to happen. You're going to have to ease your body dynamic back in the direction of health with your new behaviors.

Just like training, you'll make a little progress every single day on the path toward your goal. Those incremental steps will refine how your body works, change your cravings, and ultimately produce consistent weight loss.

Don't Forget, Don't Diet

The appetite thermometer is perhaps the closest we come to a diet in the French approach because we're asking you to keep track of your volume and how frequently you eat. But don't get too hung up on the details of the measurements or you'll slide back into the dieting mentality. Rather, focus on the point of the appestat: *You can control the quantity and quality of the food your body asks for.*

That basic fact is a freedom and a joy, because you don't have to be driven to unhealthy behaviors. Everything you will need to own your own health is within your reach, and this step gives you the tools so you can see the changes happen, quantitatively if you want, over time.

When you're adding your delicious ender to your meal, focus on the flavor and the enjoyment of the process. This will keep it in a healthy perspective. If you look at it like a magic hunger-be-gone pill, it will not work well because you'll eat too fast and drive up the amount you need to achieve the same effect. Keep it luscious and use it to practice your sensual eating. That way it will remain healthy for you and you can enjoy it each day.

CHEAT SHEET: Eat All You Want (You'll Just Want Less)

The ender is a lovely metaphor for the entire French style of eating. It represents the love of good food, the exchange of quantity for quality, the health benefits of eating small, and the importance of enjoying what you have in front of you. The promise of this technique is that you can finally own your own health and sculpt your cravings in a positive way. As a result, you'll spend more time with less food, enjoy good nutrition without going overboard, and the calories you avoid will provide weight loss without even trying.

- Wait ten minutes after your meal, and then have an ender: cheese, chocolate, nuts, tea, or coffee.

- Keep the portion small: for cheese or chocolate, only two thumbs, no more. For a liquid ender, only sip from a small cup.
- Make your enders last as long as possible.

When Finding Your Appetite Thermometer Threshold
- Add up your portions in the way that makes sense to you. Just be consistent every time.
- Eat at consistent mealtimes.
- Foods with natural levels of fiber, fat, and protein will make it easier to end grazing.
- Map your between-meal hunger blip—when it starts and how long it lasts.

The Results You're Looking For

IMMEDIATELY
- You will go longer between meals before getting hungry.
- You will understand (and learn to control) the between-meal blip.

WITHIN A WEEK
- You will have trained your physiology to be free from the constant expectation of more and more food.

WITHIN TWO WEEKS
- You will have a good sense of how much your body craves and know how to dial down the appetite thermometer threshold.

WITHIN A MONTH
- Your body will have lost your between-meal hunger blip.
- You will find yourself at the next meal and you won't really be all that hungry.

HOMEWORK: END BETWEEN-MEAL SNACKING

1. Try different enders to see which one you enjoy the most:
   a. Foods such as cheese, dark chocolate, or nuts.
   b. Drinks such as a small coffee or tea.

2. When you try these enders, note the one that takes you between meals without hunger. You may find that nuts like almonds work the best because they have fats, fiber, and calcium!

3. Track your appetite thermometer reading:

    a. Take your reading every day for the first week.

    b. Then compare all later readings with that weekly average.

Determine what your own physiology needs in order to lower portions at the plate, and increase the time between meals before you get hungry.

Living a Life You Love

Imagine a life of enjoyment, where you're not owned by your job, run by your schedule, or whipped into constant motion by the hamster wheel of overachievement. This, of course, is a description of the entire French approach to life, with long lunches of delicious foods and much longer summer vacations. Great for them, you say, but we live on a different cultural planet. Can you even conceive of the U.S. government mandating a minimum of five weeks of vacation for everyone—to hang out with your family, go somewhere together, and enjoy the summer?

When I first learned about this French tradition, I couldn't believe it. What do you mean they all go on vacation for more than a month? Two hours for lunch—what can you do sitting around for that long? What about getting work done? What about going to your job? But the French believe that living is the point of life and working is just a means to that end. Our American work ethic seems to dictate the opposite: The point of living is to work at your job, and life is just a vehicle for it.

There's more to the French lifestyle than baguettes, Brie, and Bordeaux. If you really want to get the French Don't Diet results, it's important to commit to living a more relaxed lifestyle. More and more evidence shows that stress is just as harmful to your weight as it is to your heart. Although we all crave relaxation, stress can actually be quite difficult to give up, as being perpetually busy has been so continually reinforced by our culture. But you don't have to give into that! You can live your life and love it, too, by being more than the sum of your schedules and errands—even if you can't take a longer lunch break tomorrow or increase your number of vacation days.

Part Three, "Living a Life You Love," provides this framework for you to complete the French approach to weight loss. We'll start right at home, with a return to the family dinner table. I'll show you in Step 8 why many of our health problems have emerged as a result of losing this tradition, and how to instill a social eating atmosphere that helps reduce your portions, and thereby your weight.

Step 9 moves away from the table and into the stresses of your day, which frustrate your mind, body, and any efforts at controlling your weight problems on psychological and physiological levels. This step provides easy daily solutions to handle your agenda overload. You don't have to eliminate stress altogether, just deal with it more effectively.

Sure, exercise can be a wonderful stress reliever—but for many of us, the thought of getting up early to drag ourselves to the gym just adds more anxiety to the day. Step 10 will turn your approach to exercise upside down when we look at the French alternative. When you think of southern Europeans, you don't immediately think of them as fitness buffs—and that's because they're not. Yes, they are fit, but no, they don't really exercise. The reason they can avoid this comes down to a fundamental distinction—the difference between activity and exercise. Step 10 gives you plenty of both to choose from.

The lesson from the French is about living a life of moderation, because anything taken to an extreme will be unhealthy for you. This includes your food, your exercise, and even your work, and is the real message of Part Three, embodied best as *joie de vivre*.

Return to the Family Table

One evening after just a few weeks in Lyon, our family was driving home, tired and hungry. We were definitely ready for dinner, but the prospect of cooking a meal after we got home seemed like a huge burden. I found myself longing for local fast food restaurants— if only I could have just whipped through the Arby's drive-thru for a five-for-five family meal deal. . . .

Fortunately, we just didn't have that option. So we dug through the refrigerator, found some onions and leftover chicken for a stir-fry with broiled potatoes, olive oil, and rosemary. We had some plums in the fridge, too, which we sliced up and drizzled with a bit of cream and brown sugar for dessert. The entire meal took about ten minutes for my wife and me to prepare. As dinner was served, it occurred to me that it actually would have taken us longer to stand in line back at our local Arby's!

And, because we made that meal and ate on plates, we all shared it together at the table. No one whisked their individual plastic containers off to the couch to watch TV or to play a video game. That's how we were forced (at least encouraged) by the culture around us to start eating real food, and sitting down as a family when we ate. After doing this for only a little while, we realized how easy and pleasant it is to eat well and eat together.

One of the first casualties in the stress-filled life is the family table.

On the priority scale, it gets relegated below appointments, activities, re-runs, and even the whims of kids who would just rather eat alone in their rooms. The problem is twofold: the perception that you don't have the time to make the family meal work and the lack of urgency for it because people don't understand how much it matters for their weight and health.

As it had been for me, this is one of the biggest challenges our PATH clients face—but if you commit to it, it has fantastic benefits. As one of our PATH participants, Carla Burns, later told me, "This way of eating *can* fit into the American lifestyle. As a family, we've made mealtime a priority (no TV or other distractions while eating). We still have pizza night every Friday, but we make it ourselves—my four-year-old daughter loves to help Mommy make pizza.

"My doctor is pleased with this approach, as my cholesterol and blood pressure levels are great. I've lost those difficult last few pounds (seven to be exact) and my gastro problems have disappeared. Best of all, I'm passing on healthy habits to our young daughter—she actually likes vegetables!"

Remember when this kind of family eating environment was the rule and not the exception? A study by the YMCA and the White House, released in 2000, showed that one in four parents eat with their families fewer than four times per week, and one in ten eat together only one time or less for any given week. Remember when the meal was about family and friends and not about grabbing a cereal bar as you wave to your spouse or kids on your way out the door? We were thinner back then. Remember that?

Family and the Family Table

"Frequency of family meals was inversely associated with tobacco, alcohol, and marijuana use; low grade point average; depressive symptoms; and suicide involvement" (Eisenberg, 2004).

SCIENCE-TO-ENGLISH TRANSLATION

It's not just about the food. Family meals help safeguard you and your kids.

The French, as well as many other Mediterranean cultures, have not (yet) lost the tradition of eating at the family table. It's the norm for them to come together for most meals, rather than fracturing meal-times into the isolation of individual rooms and TV shows.

I know that daily family meals may still sound tough to fit into your life—we're all busy—but take a step back and think about what I'm asking you to do compared to a fad diet regime that urges you to fol-low an artificial "food plan" or cut out entire food groups altogether. Sit down with your family or friends for your meals and make the same commitment in your day that you would for any other scheduled appointment. It's the most important set of relationships you'll ever cultivate.

But what does eating with others at the table have to do with losing weight?

The Top 5 Reasons the Family Table Is Good for Weight Loss

1. *Better nutrition.* For adults, the loss of the family table is a ter-rible absence that affects more than just the relationship of par-ents and their kids. Nutrition science research very clearly shows how it translates into adult weight problems as well. A 2003 study by Dr. Kerri Boutelle concluded that when we eat at the table—rather than in front of a screen, or in the car, or walking around—we tend to eat healthier foods.

   Specifically, the more you eat at the family table, the more you exchange faux foods for real foods. Dr. Dianne Neumark-Sztainer (also in 2003) found that the "frequency of family meals was positively associated with intake of fruits, vegetables, grains, and calcium-rich foods and negatively associated with soft drink consumption."

   This is very easy math: Greater nutrition equals lower weight problems.

2. *Natural portion control.* Because you're eating with people around you, you end up talking with them during the meal. This

alone can slow you down, which gives your body's satiety signals a chance to catch up to your eating pace and let you know when you're satisfied. People who eat with others are much less likely to become stuffed than those who eat alone.

Talking during the meal also discourages you from stuffing your mouth with food. When you're alone at the red light, in your private little car, it's easy to fill your cheek pockets with food before the light turns green. This is a recipe for overeating, of course, and something that doesn't happen as much when others are around.

3. *Preventing disordered eating.* Normally, a commitment to eating at the family table means that you have to schedule a time in your busy life to have the meal. This is wonderful for your weight, because it tends to be at a predictable time each day. And regular mealtimes, it turns out, are associated with a decrease in bad eating behaviors such as gobbling, passive overconsumption, and poor food choices that all encourage weight problems. Thus, according to the 2004 study by Neumark-Sztainer, the first defense against the disruptive habits of disordered eating may be the regular meal patterns of the family table.

4. *Social reinforcement.* Dr. Bruce Rabin is the medical director of the Healthy Lifestyle Program at the University of Pittsburgh Medical Center. We were talking over coffee, and he informed me that he felt the single biggest reason that dieters fail comes down to a lack of social support. This is another reason, incidentally, that the simple calories-in, calories-out idea just doesn't work in the real world. You have got to have help around you, role models, and friends along the way.

Eating with a group, especially when you're using the healthy eating habits we've learned here, is a perfect reinforcement for those new behaviors. Because, even if you don't talk to others around you about your habits, you can still notice those who are thin (eating as you are) and those who are not (gobbling their food).

5. *Help your kids.* I know this book is not about childhood obesity, but this is such an important issue, and there's very strong evidence that the family table is a perfect solution. When kids eat alone, they have no role models for how to eat well and eat moderately, no guidance for relating to others, no direction for carrying on a basic conversation. They are left to figure out these skills as best they can.

In fact, in a recent survey, overweight children ate dinner in front of the TV 50 percent of the time, compared to 35 percent of the time for normal weight children. And that's because eating at the family table promotes good nutrition and a moderate eating pace (as mentioned above). However, it also avoids the problem of passive overconsumption that we talked about in Step 4.

When you and your family eat together every day, kids learn the simple rules of eating well by example, how to be social, and how to take their time with their food. That's why this is not only important for kids and the family unit, it's also a key reason the French are so successful at eating well and staying thin throughout their lives.

How to Eat at the Family Table

1. *Stop before you start.* When you return to the family table, remember that no one eats until all are served and ready to begin. The very act of waiting—even though there's food right there in front of you—is wonderful practice to emphasize the importance of eating together. The people around you are your main concerns, not mindless consumption. When you all wait to be served, and all start together, these priorities are reinforced.

2. *Eat in courses.* Likewise, if you have more than one course, everyone must finish eating the first one before the next is served. This emphasizes the very same lesson: The meal is about more than your personal hunger, it's about social sharing as well.

3. *People watch.* The practice of noticing how others eat is another wonderful strategy that gets you out of your au gratin potatoes and forces you to attend to something else. Paying attention to others' habits also leads to the inevitable comparison: How do their eating habits compare to your own? What a perfect reminder to take your time, eat small, plan on seconds, and enjoy your food! And the result is that you prevent overeating and lose weight.

4. *Have a slow race.* When it's just our family around the table at home, we play a speed-eating game. Except, at our table, it's a race to see who's the *last* one done. And you can't cheat by leaving one little nibble and then loitering while everyone else finishes, or wait until all are almost done and then plopping a little more on your plate. My daughter Grace taught me these little tricks of the trade! Remember, make sure your meals are at least twenty minutes long.

5. *The family table for singles.* What do you do if you live alone? If you are single, it's almost a contradiction in terms for you to eat at the "family table." But even then, you can create the same atmosphere of success by applying these healthy principles to your life.

   • *Start with high expectations by serving yourself wonderful high-quality foods.* Buy fresh bread, organic veggies, and the best cuts of meat. When you enjoy them at a delicious pace, you control your portions and realize what a special gift it is you've given yourself.

   • *Make your eating environment pleasant.* Another wonderful way to treat yourself as well as you deserve is to take the time to set the table. Create an enjoyable space around you. You don't have to clean the house and mop the floors for every meal, just make sure your eating area is neat and uncluttered. Use real dishes, light a candle or two, and put on some agreeable music. The atmosphere really does matter, because the care you take in preparation reflects how well you take care of yourself. Make it nice and you'll enjoy meals more, feel better, spend more time with meals, and eat less in the process.

- *Take an author to dinner.* Chose a book by your favorite writer to be your dinner companion. Read it only at dinner, put your fork down to read between bites, and make your meal last a graciously long time. Eating while reading tends to make us eat slower, but eating in front of the TV encourages overconsumption.

- *Take takeout out of the box.* When you're home alone, it can be tempting to eat from your lap while watching reruns. Even if you're having takeout (and make sure it's real, not faux food!), always remove your chicken from the bucket, your Hunan shrimp from the carton, and your pizza from the box. Serve them on plates and you'll control your portions.

- *Eat with friends.* The more people you eat with, the better the atmosphere. You can either have them bring their own dishes already cooked or bring the raw materials and help you put things together on the spot. This gets all your friends together and encourages them to try new and interesting foods. In graduate school, we had a "wretched excess" gathering of friends where we all brought wonderful foods to someone's house and shared them together. It is good fun, good friends, good food.

❦ PEOPLE ON THE PATH

Dear Dr. Clower,

I am a type 2 diabetic. My diabetes was under control with diet and exercise until I became pregnant in February 2005. The doctors put me on insulin and a special diet that did nothing for my wellbeing and my already overweight body, and only made my blood sugars worse and my insulin needs higher. I went back to your French lifestyle plan and immediately saw results. I am now able to enjoy my pregnancy without having to take shots of insulin. I am also going to eat this way throughout my pregnancy, to help me keep my blood sugars under control.

Last night, at our family dinner table, I watched my daughter put one noodle at a time on her spoon, thinking how a year ago I would have been telling her to hurry up. I used to get frustrated with the way my daughter eats. I thought she was trying to be a mouse by nibbling things to death. Then I read about your approach, and I realized that she'd had it right all along. I immediately stopped telling her to eat faster, take bigger bites, and so on. I look at her now, taking her dainty little bites, and I think, "Yes, this is how it's supposed to be."

Now, we relax at mealtimes. I just marvel at how natural this way of eating/way of life is for children who haven't been messed up by their environment. I am enjoying retraining myself to the natural way of eating. And, by the way, I have never so enjoyed the process of losing thirty-plus pounds as I have on this approach.

Thank you so much. This IS the good life!

—Melissa F.

Late-Night Eating: The Physiology of a Myth

Efforts to keep from overeating can be frustrated by your schedule. One particular stumble happens when you work beyond the traditional time for dinner and get home late (after eight, say). What to do then? Everyone "knows" you'll get fat if you eat late at night. Right?

Eat late (begins the idea), and you'll get fat because you put food in your stomach too close to bedtime. So when you do go to sleep, the meal just lays there and ultimately turns straight into fat. That lazy food.

Although this sounds plausible, it is, in fact, a myth.

The reason comes back to physiology. You know how your fingers, toes, and nose are the first to freeze in bitter cold winter weather? That's because your body is brilliantly adaptable, responding to cold temperatures by cutting off blood flow from your periphery and keeping it in close to your core where it's vitally needed.

The same rerouting of blood happens on a much larger scale depending on your emotional state. When you're stressed, your body also diverts blood (like it does when it's cold). But in this case, it goes to the areas that (it thinks) you most need it. So picture yourself walking in the woods, and you accidentally bump into a snake that's now ready to sink its poisonous fangs into your exposed leg. It's none too pleased, and you're not having a blast either.

At this, your body immediately red-alerts blood to the brain, lungs, and muscles so you can bolt out of there in a flash. At the same time, it sends blood away from your viscera (gut) because who cares about digesting food when you've got a snake to escape from. Pupils dilate and breathing quickens. This is called the "fight or flight" (or sympathetic) response of your body. No digestion happening here.

However, when you're relaxed and calm and reasonably free from snakes, your body switches gears by routing blood away from the areas needed to run screaming into the woods. Instead, the blood goes into your visceral organs for digestion. In other words, your body associates digestion with your sense of calm. Thus, you digest your food best when you're at rest. This is just basic physiology.

So why do we feel like we need to eat and then do something to "work it off"? Or eat on the run? This is completely contrary to our body dynamic and at odds with the practices of other cultures without obesity problems. The skinny people eat late at night all the time.

In France, you can't even get a table before eight P.M. The doors don't even open. Dottie and I were in Paris for our anniversary one year. Mom was with the kids, so we had a warm April evening to ourselves, and our only task was to find the quaintest nook in Paris for our meal. The mistake we made, however, was to start out around 7:15. *No restaurants were open!*

Walk, walk, walk. We were getting good and hungry and Dottie's heels were not loving the irregular cobblestones. We finally found a place around eight that was still setting up. They looked at us as if we were solicitors (or worse . . . tourists). But they let us sit, very alone at first, as they got ready for the diners who actually knew when dinner was supposed to start.

Eating late at night is what all the Mediterranean cultures do. And it certainly doesn't cause the 60 million healthy French people to gain weight. Their food doesn't just "lay there," it's being digested. In fact, your body is designed to digest your food best when you're calm and relaxed. And when are you most at peace and therefore best suited to digest your food? At night. At bedtime.

So don't feel like you must eat dinner early or all is lost. It's an urban legend.

Restaurants and the Portions Arms Race

What about when you go out to eat? As our obesity rate has risen, so has the percentage of meals eaten at restaurants. This is not just a co-incidence, and brings up yet another French paradox. The French, of course, are famous for their restaurants, large and small, in every village, town, and city—and they visit them often! But their restaurants don't harm their health, as ours seem to do. How in the world could that be?

For one thing, much of the food served in American restaurants (particularly at the fast-food chains) is faux food, and therefore horrid for your health. But heaped on top of the faux-food factor is the portion problem. What almost all our restaurants do wrong is serve forklift-worthy portions. This reflects the average increase in plate size from eight to fourteen inches over the past twenty years. Individual serving sizes have expanded, too: a typical order of french fries in the 1980s was 2.4 ounces, compared to today's 6.9-ounce serving with 610 calories!

Why we have such enormous restaurant serving sizes was always confusing to me, until I was invited to speak for the World Presidents' Organization in Scottsdale, Arizona. My host happened to own a chain of steak restaurants. On my first day, we were chatting away about food and health, and when I mentioned "portions" he perked up. "We serve *huge* portions at my restaurants," he boasted, visibly pleased.

This position made no sense to me. If you're the restaurant owner, why on earth would you want to serve too much food? Doesn't this just needlessly add costs? Aren't you losing money on this strategy?

I brought up this little irony, and he just shook his head at my green-horn question. "My restaurants aren't the only ones around," he drawled. "I gotta compete with all them other steak houses in driving distance. If the store up the road's got larger portions than me, I gotta match them or it'll get around that I don't give enough beef for the buck!"

I got his drift. If you're working in a competitive "volume equals value" world, you have to meet this demand or you'll go out of business. If your competitors crank up the portion volume, you've got to do it, too. If they have big plates, you have to have bigger plates.

It's a portions arms race.

But we can't just blame the restaurants for the quantity or quality of their food. The recent trend is to sue fast-food restaurants for serving food that contributes to weight and health problems. Yet we no longer have an excuse—we know what we're getting when we walk in the door. And there's nothing at all *wrong* with eating at restaurants that serve good food—especially if you keep from overdoing it.

Everyone contributes to the expanding portion problem—not just businesses, but consumers as well. In fact, restaurants just reflect the demand. If consumers judged the quality of their food on the taste, texture, and aroma instead of just size, the competitive ratcheting up of portions would be less of a problem than it is now.

Whatever the cause, restaurant portion sizes do help fuel our obesity epidemic. Two researchers who've done wonderful work on this are Dr. Barbara Rolls, author of *Volumetrics,* and Dr. Marion Nestle, author of *Food Politics.* They've consistently shown that the typical wheelbarrow portions do in fact produce overconsumption. That's because the added calories on your plate are not even noticed and do nothing to decrease the amount you eat at later meals.

What to Avoid When Eating Out

Have you ever seen an all-you-can-eat buffet in France? I don't think so, unless it was put there as a tourist trap. This is the epitome of the difference between our eating cultures. All you can eat, for us, is a gorge fest where the very point is to make the meal "worth it" by eating your body weight in food. It's not about enjoyment, it's about excess.

"All you can eat," for the French, means you eat until you're satisfied. Then you stop.

The problem with harmful eating behavior like the buffet binge is that it becomes your default pattern that's very hard to break. And as we've seen, if it does become your normal unconscious mode of eating, you're in trouble. You may eat in control for a little while when you're concentrating on it, but sooner or later your old ways will kick back in and you'll return to the same disordered eating habits.

What you want is exactly the opposite—eating instincts that make you naturally gravitate toward eating less, not more. Each step we've covered so far trains your physiology to expect smaller portions on the plate and fewer between-meal snacks. These behavioral controls handle your eating habits for you over the long term, even when you're not thinking about them. So don't work against your own efforts; avoid the all-you-can-eat buffet.

Some Basic Guidelines for Eating Out

Remember the rules from previous steps: avoid faux foods, eat small bites, take your time, eat in courses, sip your drinks, have an ender.

1. Freebie appetizers like the bread and oil served before your meal can be treacherous. They come when you're still hungry, so think of them as something *you will taste, not eat.* This is a good time to practice serving less than you're hungry for and leaving a little on your plate even when you're still hungry. This is the restaurant equivalent of planning on seconds and solving the clean-your-plate problem, all at the same time. But if you have a hard time controlling yourself here, don't get the appetizer at all. Otherwise, it's a recipe for overconsumption.

2. Often, one solution for eating small is to order your meal from the appetizer menu. However, restaurants have long ago caught on to this trick by making the size and price of these selections little

different from those on the main menu. But when you're traveling, and cannot bring the Styrofoam container home, it's still the best way to control the portions they're heaping on you.

3. When you eat with others, order fewer plates than there are people at the table, and share them among yourselves. This allows you to taste a variety of flavors, and works particularly well with Asian cuisine and when you're eating with family members and close friends.

4. Some restaurants serve half portions. If you find one that does, you should reinforce their good behavior by eating there!

5. A few places might offer the "menu"—the practice is commonplace in France, but can be seen as hoity-toity elsewhere. It's simply a series of courses all linked together. The portions of each course are smaller, and they're served over time. This definitely helps you control volume and extends the length of your meal. So if you find a restaurant that serves its courses in a menu, give it a try!

6. If your salad and main meal come to the table at the same time, eat your salad second. We normally eat the salad first, but that just means your main course will be getting colder by the bite! This causes you to rush through the salad to get to the entree. The solution is to save the naturally cold plate, the salad, until you are done with the hot plate.

7. When you're eating alone, can't share a plate, and aren't on the road, make it a normal practice to have the waiter bring a to-go box with your meal. Before you begin, put half of your portion away before you even start. If it's in the box already, you won't eat it, and then you know you'll have plenty left for lunch tomorrow. This puts you in complete control of your portions.

Restaurants don't have to be hazardous to your health, but you do have to be ready for the amount of food you know they're going to serve you. Cut it in half, split it among friends, and definitely plan on ordering less than you're hungry for. That way you can have a wonderful lunch or night out without having to worry about it harming your weight and health.

Troubleshooting the Family Table

❦ *Problem: An irregular eating schedule.*
   Solution: Keep consistency where you can.

Many people who have work schedules that vary week by week simply cannot establish a routine for those around them, particularly when that person is the one who usually does the cooking! That leaves the rest of the family to "fend for themselves," which can be a disaster for their eating choices and habits. And if you are the one with the irregular schedule, you can find yourself resorting to whatever you can find at the 7-Eleven on your way home.

Keep your main meals in the general vicinity of the same time. In other words, even if your breakfast isn't at 8:05 exactly and you have to eat at 9:15, that's okay. When this happens, you've got to try to get back to your normal scheduled eating times as soon as you can. So, for example, if you have breakfast at 9:15 you'll still eat at 12:00 for lunch (if possible). But bear in mind that your time between meals is shortened—so you won't need as much for breakfast.

Your eating environment should also be maintained, even if you aren't eating at the same time of day. If you normally eat at your kitchen table at home, or in the cafeteria at work, keep to the same basic pattern. At the very least, maintaining a consistent eating environment serves as a behavioral anchor for you and helps reinforce your healthy eating habits.

❦ *Problem: No support from family and friends.*
   Solution: Have them join you—or distance yourself.

By making eating social again, we really introduce a double-edged sword. It's wonderful to share your meal with others, but it can become difficult when those around you are not supportive of your efforts to eat small and take your time at the meal. Kids whine and spouses may tease about your lower portions.

If you can remain uninfluenced by the counterproductive eating habits of those around you, that's fantastic. Otherwise, you need to enroll them into eating this way so you don't backslide into their harmful routines.

Tina, a woman in the PATH Healthy Eating Curriculum, related how her husband would always comment on her small portions: "You makin' love to that or you gonna eat it?" She tried to persuade him to eat this way with her, but ultimately couldn't slow him down. He would be done by the time she was only halfway through her meal. So she ended up having to eat in two phases: the first part with her husband and the second part after he'd cleared out. Actually, she said the peace and quiet of the second half . . . wasn't half bad.

Meryl, a woman from another PATH course, had a similar problem in that her husband brought home faux-food snacks to eat right in front of her as a taunt. Meryl told me she couldn't be in the same room with the Oreos, so "that was my cue that I needed to go upstairs for my meditation/relaxation time."

These examples illustrate the different ways of handling this problem: Enroll those around you, adapt to their habits without giving up your own, or just take yourself out of the environment.

⚜ *Problem: Cooking for one.*
Solution: Keep it interesting.

Eating at the family table sounds wonderful in principle. But if you're alone and make a pot of spaghetti (especially as you learn to eat small again), you could have that vat sitting in your fridge for weeks until you are sick of that sauce!

Another issue that arises with single people who cook for themselves is that they get bored with their food. Once they've made their best two or three dishes, they're faced with them over and over and just don't want to eat them anymore.

The first solution is to never make the whole recipe. Especially now that you're learning how to control your consumption, you've got to "downshift" and cut everything you make into thirds. This is the equivalent of serving less than you think you need. That said, some things may be made in bulk, such as chili or soup, as these will freeze and rewarm nicely.

To prevent boredom in the kitchen, take cooking classes. Literally spice up your life. Start with the standard ones—French and Italian—and then branch out. Learn to cook with spices you're not used to: Thai with spicy sweet coconut, Indian with curry, or even Japanese cuisine. There are so many options, and when you are taking the course, you can't go wrong.

Don't Forget, Don't Diet

Zoom out. Stop focusing so closely on the minutiae that you can't see what's really important for your weight and health. Macromolecules are important, but bigger issues affect how much of them you consume, from the top down: social eating habits, the people around you, the eating environment. All these influence your overall food volume, and therefore can determine your weight.

Have you noticed how this aspect, the human element of eating, never gets covered by standard dieting methods? Rather, you are encouraged only to account for fats and carbs, and so end up eating quickly, and alone. Your consumption rises, causing calories to increase, and you become another of the 95 percent of people for whom diets fail. And, unfortunately, many end up blaming themselves for a failure that wasn't their fault. It was the method that failed them by forgetting the social importance of eating.

So here's some advice for losing weight by living the French lifestyle without dieting: Eat well, and take your time with your family and friends to get to know them through each meal. When this becomes the priority it needs to be, you will find that the process takes longer, you enjoy it more, you eat less, and your weight and health are the final beneficiaries.

CHEAT SHEET: THE FAMILY TABLE

The atmosphere around the family table fosters healthy food choices, controlled consumption, and a better relationship with food. This same comfortable atmosphere can be applied at home, in a restaurant, and for single people as well.

To create an atmosphere of healthy eating:
- Turn off all technology except the answering machine.
- Schedule your time to make the family table a priority.
- Avoid the all-you-can-eat buffet.
- Treat yourself right with high-quality foods.
- Treat yourself right by setting up a nice eating space.

The Results You're Looking For

IMMEDIATELY
- You will love the eating environment you create.
- You will find yourself more relaxed at the table.
- You will talk more with those around you.

WITHIN TWO WEEKS
- You will eat slower and enjoy it more.
- You will control portions at home and at restaurants.

WITHIN A MONTH
- Your family will have gotten so used to your new eating habits that they will be perfectly normal and accepted.
- You'll feel comfortable enough to never have to worry about overconsuming in restaurants.

HOMEWORK: SOCIAL EATING

1. Schedule your meals to include others as part of your commitment to your weight and health.
2. If you live alone, prepare the table so it's an inviting space.
3. If you live alone, take an author to dinner.

4. Always people watch! Notice their eating habits in relation to your own.
5. Encourage those around you to eat small and race to be the last one finished.
6. Always bring something home from the restaurant.
7. When eating with friends or family, spend more time talking than eating.

Find Your Peace

F rance from 12:00 P.M. to 2:30 P.M. is a beautiful thing. The clatter of forks on plates and the chatter of friends over food just makes you want to sit for a while. When you're in this environment, you're drawn into relaxing. And there's nothing to do about it but enjoy yourself, because other businesses basically close—you're expected to take a break through the lunch period. It sounds wonderful and it is, but it actually takes some getting used to.

Imagine my dilemma of starting a new job in a new country, wanting to impress the world with my industry and productivity. In the first few overeager days, I'd run back from lunch at 12:30 to get more work done. But it didn't take many iterations of marching back to my desk through the empty echoing halls before I realized that no one else was there—except those few heading off to eat a little late.

No one—the software specialists, the engineers, the secretaries—would be returning until around 2:30 P.M., so if I needed anything at all I'd have to go back out to the cafeteria or the break room and find them there. They were never much help, though, at easing my work-related angst, so I eventually realized that I might as well just relax, sit down, chat with them, and enjoy myself. It was excruciating until the moment it hit me that I needed to just calm down for a second. Moreover, I discovered that I actually got just as much done as I ever had before!

Although they loathe the workaholic mentality, the French are still very productive people. They're just much better at pacing themselves: They work hard in the morning, relax for a couple of hours, and then work hard in the afternoon until about 6:30. In fact, learning theory shows that taking a break between bouts of industry can actually be the most efficient use of your time. When you're engaged in any mental or physical task, sustained effort without a pause soon becomes counterproductive as you lose your edge, make mistakes, and get less work accomplished in the time you do have.

Thus, the way to really improve your performance is actually to *not perform for a while*. Your brain essentially needs to rest for periods of time between bouts of effort (be they math, or memory, or learning a new motor skill). So do yourself a favor and take a break. As soon as you let yourself stop for a while and direct your attention elsewhere, you'll find that you're much more engaged (and engaging) when you return.

Throughout this book we've talked about high-quality foods replacing high-quantity eating, but the same is just as true for your life. You can speed through your day nonstop to get more and more done until you collapse in bed, but you'll actually get as much accomplished by taking a breather between quality, focused jags of productivity—and you certainly won't burn out as fast.

Stressful Eating

"Stressors and emotion-focused coping were found to be associated with low self-esteem, which in turn was strongly associated with disturbed eating attitudes. Stressors were also directly related to disturbed eating attitudes" (Fryer, 1997).

SCIENCE-TO-ENGLISH TRANSLATION

One hundred percent fat-free, carb-free stress produces disordered eating, which produces weight problems.

Are you ready for the biggest secret of the French approach? To be thin, healthy, and energetic you need to enjoy your life: Sleep well, laugh out loud, take time to play, and mentally relax. These factors are critical. Compelling scientific data show why the gracious ease of the French approach actually works better in the long term, and a big reason for this comes down to stress reduction.

Each day, we drive ourselves into a harried frenzy that can cascade into weight gain, high blood pressure, heart disease, and even depression. That's because living a life out of emotional balance causes blood sugar swings, which turn into insulin instabilities, which turn into fat storage and in some cases, diabetes. These physiological effects of stress provide another explanation for the success of the French approach, which frees them from this slippery slope of health problems. But you can do this, too, by handling the stress your life; otherwise, the molecules you happen to micromanage will be irrelevant.

Chronic stress can make you fat.

Stress and Your Body

Stress is like wine and chocolate: beneficial in small doses and harmful in large ones. Our bodies are built to respond to stress with short bursts of energy, activity, and mental focus. These stressful situations prime you for an "on the edge" level of performance, which begins with a quick shot of adrenaline. But when prolonged, day in and day out, it becomes terrible for every system in your body. And it all starts because stress causes your physiology to think you need energy, so it produces the hormone cortisol.

What Happens to Your Muscles
In its turn, cortisol elevates and maintains blood glucose (sugar) levels by speeding up the breakdown of muscle protein into amino acids (to make more glucose). This can lead to muscle wasting.

What Happens to Your Immune System
Chronic cortisol also inhibits the immune system by decreasing the antibody and T-cell response to infections, the number of white blood cells, and even slows how long it takes a wound to heal. You get sicker easier, and stay sicker longer.

What Happens to Your Bones

Long-term stress inhibits normal bone formation, robs calcium from bones, and decreases the calcium that can be absorbed into your body. This weakens your bones, makes you more susceptible to fracture, and prevents your body from doing the normal work of bone repair.

What Happens to Your Heart

Stress is linked to heart attacks. That much is plain, although the reasons why are only now being discovered, with several important leads. For example, the cortisol produced by chronic stress impairs your heart's most basic reflexes (the baroreflex sensitivity) and actually physically impairs how your arteries function. It also tends to increase the ratio of sodium to potassium in your blood—the recipe for high blood pressure. Whatever the details turn out to be, it's clear that prolonged mental stress leads to heart disease.

What Happens to Your Nervous System

Stressed individuals often become neurological patients and can suffer a range of problems from sleep deprivation to depression. Also, as your daily muscle tensions build up over days you become fatigued, even when you've not expended any excess energy. Chronic migraines are frequent and can even induce eating disorders, as noted in this 2005 research by Dr. Sandra Sassaroli: "In female individuals, stress might bring out a previously absent association between some psychological predisposing factors for eating disorders and an actual desire or plan to lose weight. *Such a finding suggests that stress may stimulate behaviors related to eating disorders in a predisposed personality.*"

Science-to-English translation? Stress can induce eating disorders where there were none before.

What Happens to Your Weight

Stress does everything wrong for your health and weight. It stimulates the hunger drive psychologically and physiologically so you eat more, but it also causes blood to be routed away from the digestive organs at the same time. It inhibits gastric secretions and may exacerbate ulcers. Thus, you are eating more but digesting it all very poorly! Even worse, stress hormones have recently been shown to cause your body to preferentially store fat in your abdominal region.

Not only are you hungry for more food more often—digesting it poorly and storing your food as fat around your stomach—your eating pace quickens and the size of your bite increases. This quickly leads to overconsumption.

Once you understand these physical effects of stress, another French paradox clears up: "How can France be such a productive country when they take so much time off?" Our basic physiology explains it by showing the physical benefits of moderation, the long-term health that comes from periodically taking time off, and the mental clarity afforded by hopping off the hamster wheel once in a while.

If we're going to get these benefits, too, we need techniques to decrease stress on a daily basis in our own culture. So practice the lessons below and you'll kick off a cascade of health effects behind the metabolic scenes. Your cortisol levels will lower, your immune system will strengthen, your blood sugar will stabilize, and your weight will drop. And all you have to do to move in this healthy direction is to relax.

⚜ PEOPLE ON THE PATH

Dear Dr. Clower,

Day 5 of "training my body." It's been so much easier than I expected. And one surprise has been the sense of something missing— familiarity. I am so familiar with my worries, frustrations, and internal chatter about what I'm eating, how much, how often, and so on. When that goes away, as it has the last couple of days, it's almost disorienting.

I sense how much easier and more familiar it might all be if our larger culture had a healthy, pleasure-based orientation to food and eating. Part of the unfamiliarity is just how alien this way of eating seems in our cultural context.

I'm stunned at how easily I've slid into the smaller portions, smaller meals, and slower eating. I have resisted those things for a long time. Now I find I'm looking forward to sitting at the table and taking those small, conscious bites—looking forward more than I ever imagined. There's a lot that has to change to support these sane practices. Like eating before I jump in the car for an early-morning trip, instead of grabbing the food and eating it on the road. Different—and better, so far.

—Rona R.

Love Your Life Like You Love Your Food

Joie de vivre, or the joy of living, is a common French attitude. It's about being more committed to finding happiness in your ordinary daily life than being a slave to your schedule or perceptions of productivity and success. This relaxed attitude has been shown to promote heart health, low weight, and even longer lives. It's great in theory, but how do you live a life you love in the dizzy swirl of our breakneck speed culture? How do you find your peace on your terms?

Get Real

There is no difference between an authentic stress and a perceived one. In other words, you can shape your own reality. That's all nice and philosophical, but this hits home on a practical level, too. There are a million things in your life that you could spin your mental wheels worrying about, from your checkbook to your relationship to the neighbors' choice of house paint to global warming.

You have to be selective about which you choose because, as just mentioned, worry cascades into weight and health problems. Really think about the issues in your life that matter. To do this, take a sheet of paper and release your worries by writing every single one of them down—no matter how trivial. But here's how you do it. Write them down in two columns: those "worth the cortisol" and those that are not. You may be facing some big issues that you cannot escape, but you will find that most of your list falls into the "not worth the cortisol" column. Once you see them for the little things they really are, let them go and just handle them as soon as you can.

And, for those items you do have to spend some mental energy on, below are some strategies for overcoming them. These suggestions help you find your peace daily by using the very same principles we've described so far for loving your food. This is the lesson of the French diet, applied beyond your food and into your life.

Take Your Time

The French habits of healthy eating teach you to relax around your food, training you out of the sixty-miles-per-hour gobbling that becomes a superhighway to health problems. And just like you should give your food the time it deserves, the same applies to your personal relationships.

Think back to the times in your life when you really connected with your parents, spouse, or friends. This never happened when they were stone-skipping their way through tasks, leaving you feeling like item thirty-four on their list of things to do. It was when they finally stopped, sat down, and really gave you their attention. Well, when you're on the other end, remember that your time and attention are gifts you can give to the people you love, and ones you'll get back by creating the close bonds that really matter.

Focus on the people around you and the quality of your life will be enhanced—even though you may not be checking off as many things from your infinite to-do list.

- When people speak to you, you have to silence the commentary that runs in your head about what they're saying, what they're wearing, or what you'll do after they finish. Be totally present to them and what they are trying to communicate. This is not always easy; it's a skill you'll need to practice.

- Stop, drop, or enroll. If you're in the middle of something, just stop what you're doing and turn your attention to the person in front of you. If you cannot, let them know you're almost done, finish it up, and then turn your attention to the person in front of you. If you cannot (like when you're cooking), enroll them to help you!

- Plan on doing nothing. When they get together with family and friends, some people fill their time with wall-to-wall events that are actually nothing more than an extended set of distractions. Plan on doing nothing for a time with those around you. After a while, if you find that everyone's ready to get out of the house and go do something again, it's no problem that you didn't already have an agenda planned. That's your opportunity to be spontaneous!

Taste Life with Smaller Bites

Here's the rule for our meals: Take smaller bites or you won't even taste them. When your mouth is overfull, 90 percent of the food doesn't even touch your taste buds! Instead of swallowing as much as possible all at once to get it over with, it's vital to taste what you're consuming.

The same principle applies to your daily life. Remember, life's to-do list is infinite. There will always be three more items nagging at you to get started on even before the last one is begun, so make the decision to focus your energy on the task at hand. Otherwise, you'll always be looking—and living—past the items that are right in front of you.

When we bite off more than we can chew, our body has its own way of getting our attention with the stress-related health problems that emerge from the over-scheduled life. Less is more in this case. In the same way, whenever possible, take smaller bites of life. Make your tasks, your vacations, and your schedule realistic, and therefore manageable, so you can be more present and more focused on what you're doing. This is how to savor your life every day.

- Focus on the little things. Even during the melee of the weekday, don't rush past the little kindnesses that make this spinning planet a tolerable place. Take time to pet your animals, tell someone thank you and mean it, surprise someone you care about.

- On the weekends, whenever you can, take an afternoon nap or an evening bath. These little indulgences allow you to digest the daily whir for a moment and reinforce how much more important you are than your schedule.

- Stop multitasking, so you won't ever feel as if you've got more on your plate than you can handle at any one time. Schedule your events in series, not in parallel, and you'll be more effective and be less likely to wake up one morning and find yourself completely overwhelmed with your life.

Pause Between Bites

Living in perpetual motion is exactly like eating nonstop—both lead to mindless consumption. Our habits of healthful eating teach you to put your fork down between bites, so you can reflect on what you're eating. You should do the same thing with your life.

When your schedule is packed from morning to midnight, and life is filled to capacity at every second, you certainly can't taste it. Have you ever gotten to the end of a day or month or year and thought, "What just happened here? What did I do yesterday?" Or "Where did the time go?" This happens when you try to cram too much into the limited space of your day.

Be here now, as the saying goes. Live in the present and make it a point to attend to what's right in front of you: the sights and sounds and smells and textures. To enjoy your life, you have to notice it first. And to notice it, you have to stop and give your present task your complete attention.

- *Be at peace with this math.* Your possible to-do list will never end, but your life on this planet will. It's your choice to subtract some of your errands in exchange for a little added life. There's always more to do, but you don't have to do it.

- *Plan on seconds!* Always put less on your (metaphorical) plate than you think you can accomplish. If Saturday is your cleaning day, have the whole day reserved for that. If you finish and need something else to do, you can always go back and add it on without a problem.

- *Keep some of yourself in reserve.* Everyone wants your time, and you can easily give so much of yourself that you have nothing left. Politely, firmly, let the askers know that you just can't do it. Don't lose yourself to someone else's agenda.

Your Relationship with Food Is Like Your Relationship with Life

Just as we often confuse the love of food with gluttony and value with volume, we can also conflate the love of life with busywork. Don't you know people who think they're getting the most out of life when they take on as much as possible, as though at the end of their lives they can look back at a long list of "Been there, done that"? (Got the husband, been to Grand Canyon, got the car, been to Venice, got the house, visited Great Wall, got 2.5 kids, took tennis lessons, got a promotion . . .) They march through this list as if to say, "See how much I loved my life?" But this is just like overeating an absurd amount of food and looking up as if to say, "See how much I loved my food?"

By contrast, make your life like a long, lingering love affair with dark chocolate truffles, rather than the mindless stuffing of handfuls of cheap, corn syrup "chocolates." You want your life to be a peach so pungent, so full of flavor running down your chin that it makes your mouth water to think of it, not a biggie-size bucket of dyed food products. And when you look back at your life, it will have been rich and full only if you happened to notice it. At that point, you will be satisfied.

Now here's the caveat. There are people who find joy in their type

A behavior. For those of you who could do nothing else but busily plow through your lists of things to do, and this truly gives you happiness, bless you.

The point is that you don't *have* to unplug or slow down, because loving your life is not quantitative—it doesn't matter whether you fill your day with two things or a hundred. It only matters whether you can be at peace with living the life you choose. For example, most of us cannot juggle fifty of life's batons at once (work, boss, coworkers, home, cleaning, spouse, kids, parent duties, events, pets, night school, and on and on) without getting frazzled around the edges. There are those rare few, however, who genuinely love such an environment and thrive in it. They aren't stressed by this kind of life, they're thrilled by it. But for most of us—if you don't love it, don't do it.

- *Be sensual.* Get out of your head and pay attention to the sights, sounds, smells, tastes, and textures around you. Let your eyes drift from the computer screen and really notice your world for a moment. The screen will still be there when you come back.

- *Be honest.* Be realistic with yourself about the number of items you have to do in a day. If your life feels like a blur at the end of the day, you've got to cut back. Are you really enjoying your life every day? If not, be prepared to trade in your high quantity for a little more quality.

- *Be physical.* Nothing can be such a good "reboot" as getting outside and moving around. For me, a good solid bout of physical exertion is a fantastic way to disengage my mind from the hurly-burly of the day. But even if you don't exercise, you can take a quick jaunt outside and move around for a minute on your break.

Stress-Relief Routines

The French culture makes it very easy to live a pleasant life. But we live in a society that not only doesn't offer two-hour lunch breaks and five weeks of paid vacation, it seems to pride itself on anxiety. Our unfortunately frequent response to that is to eat. Thus, we need practical strategies to cope with and even reduce the stress of everyday life.

The first and easiest way to relieve stress in your life is to simply leave time open during your day. Don't fill every minute with tasks and chores. Of course you have a normal life to lead, but you can set aside a little time—if only a few minutes—for yourself. How?

- *Delegate.* You don't have to do everything yourself. Enroll those around you in your tasks as well. Then you're a team!

- *Schedule.* Set aside time for yourself in advance, like an appointment, and stick to it.

- *Control the list.* Don't give in to extra errands sneaking into your schedule, as your to-do list expands to fit your time. Determine what you want to get done for the day, and if you accomplish it, your free time is your reward!

With these basics, you can lift yourself out of the bottomless to-do abyss and you'll do your body a favor as well. But more important is the link between your body and mind, which needs relaxing every day. Just as you clear time in your schedule, practice clearing your mind whenever you can. This gets you out of the constant mental whir of activities and worries that spin through your head and gives you a break from the stress hormones that can damage your health.

Deep Breathing—Instant Stress Relief

When we're anxious, we breathe from the chest in shorter, quicker bursts of air. When calm, we tend to breathe deeply from the stomach. But does that mean that stress causes chest breathing? Or is increased stress an effect of rapid breathing? Actually, there's no clear difference between the cause of your breathing patterns and the effect of them. Chest breathing encourages your body to have a stress response, while belly breathing encourages your body to release stress. It's another circle.

Just as your emotions influence behaviors (being stressed causes chest breathing, being calm causes belly breathing), your behaviors can also influence your emotions. Make use of this knowledge every day and control your body's stress response by practicing the healthy breathing techniques that can help lower cortisol. Once you practice them for a few weeks and make them a habit, you're in control for life.

The following breathing routine can help calm your mind and reduce your daily stress. Whenever you feel anxious, this technique will help you think more clearly and concentrate better.

1. Sit in a chair and put your left hand on your belly. Now put your right hand on the center of your chest. Inhale slowly and deeply, and focus on the movement of your hands. You want the hand on your stomach to rise and fall with your breaths, and the hand on your chest to move only slightly.

2. When you've inhaled fully, hold your breath there and slowly count to three.

3. Exhale slowly and completely to empty your lungs.

4. Repeat this 3 to 5 times, but be careful not to hyperventilate. If you feel dizzy, you've just gotten too much oxygen and you can pause.

This technique can be used absolutely anywhere: when the traffic is terrible, when you're trying to get to sleep, or when something is upsetting you.

Good Morning Meditation

This simple method can help center your mind before the maelstrom of the day. It can lower the stress hormones in your blood, train you to become less responsive to stressful events, and counteract their accumulated effects.

Meditation helps you temporarily transfer your thinking away from the whirring, worrying thoughts that permeate our minds. With this technique, you'll instead focus on a single message, rather than on your normal nagging thoughts. This makes meditation basically a neural trick (respectful apologies to meditation teachers), but a healthy one that may be perhaps the single most overlooked aspect of wellness.

1. Find a quiet place where you can sit comfortably.

2. Select a word, phrase, sound, or repetitive movement (as in tai chi, for example) to focus your attention on. Whatever you choose should have a positive meaning to you. You might try *peace, easy,* or *rest.* Focus your mind on your breath as you inhale (through your mouth or nose, it doesn't matter), and then say your word to yourself or out loud during the exhale.

3. When you begin, keep your eyes closed so you won't be distracted by the visual environment around you. (However, you might place a clock in easy view so you can peek at it if necessary to see how long you've been at it.)

4. Breathe and focus for about fifteen minutes in the morning. If, while meditating, a thought comes into your mind, don't panic and stop. Just consciously ease your attention back to your breathing and your word.

Breathe and focus using this technique at least three times per week, preferably in the morning. The more you practice relaxing your mind, the easier it will be to slip into that relaxed state. First it becomes easier to relax through the meditation period, but then you'll notice increased relaxation and peace through your day. Expect it to take anywhere from a couple of days to a couple of weeks of practice before you begin to realize how much the technique helps calm your mind. It just depends on the individual person.

Remember, letting go of stress is just like every other new habit. There's no switch that you can flip from on to off. Even though the techniques are simple, you do have to practice them to make them a steady part of your life. This is how "finding your peace" becomes easier as you go.

Yoga

Is yoga an exercise or a stress management technique? Actually, it's both. If you need a little of both and don't have the time to sign up for full contact karate *and* transcendental meditation, yoga gives you a bit of both, all at the same time. It's good for your heart, for your body, and for your mind.

In fact, it's so healthy that it is now being studied by rigorous medical scientists. In a 2004 paper, Dr. Parshad investigated the various ways yoga improves overall health. These include muscle strength, flexibility, improved circulation and oxygen uptake, as well as hormone function. And the relaxation clearly helps yoga practitioners be more resilient to stressful situations. This, in turn, helps them reduce risk factors for cardiorespiratory diseases. These wonderful benefits have been known in Eastern cultures for centuries, and are just now receiving their proper medical explanations in the West.

Laughter Lightens the Heart

Humor really does heal. In fact, decades of research has shown that humor—and the physical act of laughing—is an incredibly effective intervention for cancer patients, decreasing anxiety, boosting the immune system, and reducing stress hormones. After all, laughter has a trove of positive physiological effects such as lowering blood pressure, increasing relaxation, and perhaps even helping prevent heart disease.

So find something that makes you laugh every day. Especially when your situation provokes worry and anxiety, try to find the humor that will lighten your emotional load. Call it your cancer-prevention medicine, your heart medicine, or your immunity-boosting medicine, because that's what it is. Laugh, doctor's orders.

One day Janet, a woman in our PATH to Healthy Weight Loss course, worried to me that she had to serve on a voter registration panel, but wasn't looking forward to it. The panel was made up of people who just seemed to be perpetually grumpy. Even though it wasn't until the next week, she was already working up a good solid case of dread about it. One of her coworkers in particular was so negative about absolutely everything she said, she was sure it would make the day unbearable. And, of course, the poor poll workers are easy targets for rude people who come by and blame them for any perceived slight.

This issue was bearing down on Janet, but it's something almost everyone faces in some form or another all the time. How can you stay positive in your life in the face of boring work and the company of negative people? It's not easy, but here's what I advised for her.

1. *Negate the negative.* I coached Janet to sit as far away from the negative coworker as possible. Grumpy people are unfortunately plentiful and stuck in their ways. Always position yourself around people who are upbeat; they'll elevate your mood and naturally support your happiness and health. You can do the same thing at home by choosing comedy TV shows and radio programs. You don't have to do this all the time, just make sure to include the infectiousness of humor somewhere in your entertainment lineup.

2. *See it your way.* If her colleagues insisted on sharing their black clouds, she could mentally distance herself from them by viewing their ridiculous comments as she would a cartoon: Eeyore, Yosemite Sam, Grumpy the dwarf. These guys are all funny because they're just playing the role of the disgruntled person for the scene. For the real people in front of you, when you choose to see them as caricatures of their ugly emotions, you're more detached and less likely to take personally whatever problems they're working themselves through. In this light, their bark loses its bite.

3. *Clock out.* For those times when no voters are drifting by, Janet could take an enjoyable book to fill her time with. It wouldn't have to be funny per se, but something that would make her smile. Look for the funny, quirky, offbeat elements that are around you all the time. Do this as a commitment to a lightened spirit that helps ward off even chronically gloomy people of the world. Don't let them drag you down.

Take a Muscle Inventory

Check in with your body and you'll be able to release tension in just seconds. It takes no more than a couple minutes to make a mental survey of your muscles. It's a body scan you can do on yourself. In fact, go ahead and try this now. It helps to do this with your eyes closed.

1. *Think about your shoulder muscles.* If they're tight, let them go slack. Roll your shoulders back. They may tense up later on, but that's okay because by doing this you've broken the chronic contractions with a brief period of relaxation. See how easy that was? And it only took a few seconds!

2. *Focus on your face.* Now take a brief muscular inventory from the neck up. Start at your neck muscles, especially at the base of your skull and then slowly move around to beneath your chin. Think about whether they are tightened up, one at a time, and consciously relax them. Now move to the biggest cause of tension headaches, the muscles of your face. Think about the tightness you experience around your eyes, then in your forehead and finally down to your jaw muscles. Let them go slack, one at a time.

3. *Down to your toes.* With the same procedure, move to the muscles along your neck and upper back, arms, and legs. At each stage, check for tightness and relax the muscles for a few seconds, long enough to release the tension before continuing. You'll find the most productive area you have to work on will be around your upper back, which is the region that gets scrunched up when you hunch your shoulders.

Take your muscle inventory daily and two important things happen. First, relaxation becomes a more natural part of your day as you begin to sense the strain that builds up in your shoulders and around your eyes before it turns into a tension headache. And *once you begin to notice* muscle tension within your normal day, you'll be more likely to relax your muscles—it becomes automatic. At that point you have a lifetime solution that heads off stress before it can affect you physically.

The second thing that happens when you practice relaxing your muscles daily is that you tap into the relationship between your body and mind. While it's true that mental stress causes physical stress, chronic physical stress also causes mental stress. It goes both ways. That's why, when you relax the muscles of (especially) your face and neck, your overall level of anxiety is reduced as well.

You've probably heard the old saying that it's the little things that matter most. Taking care of your muscle tension periodically through the day is perhaps the easiest, quickest thing you can do to handle chronic stress in your life.

Writing

Venting can be an important stress-relieving outlet for many people. But the problem with venting is that you're usually doing it *at* someone— not a good idea. However, the technique I want to show you really helps you vent, but in a productive way . . . by writing.

Don't worry, you don't have to be a good writer. And don't worry about getting the words, spelling, or grammar perfect (your scribblings won't be seen by anyone but you). But by consistently venting your thoughts on the page, you'll find that the effects can be dramatic. To do this, follow these simple rules:

1. With a notebook and pen, find a quiet spot where you'll have about fifteen minutes of time to yourself.

2. The only rule is that you need to write continuously. You don't have to write fast, just keep the words flowing. And it doesn't matter what you choose to write about either, because you're simply venting onto the page and the subjects will come out on their own. If you run out of topics to write about, restate what you've already written down. Just keep writing something for the entire fifteen minutes.

3. When you're done, tear up the page and throw it away, so your journal can never be seen. You can tell it anything.

You will find that, as with everything, this process gets easier as you continue. At first you may have to repeat what you've already written a few times, but by the second and third attempt you'll be able to spill all the pent-up thoughts right out on the page.

Keep in mind that your venting doesn't have to be negative. Positive venting can be very liberating when you write your gratitude, hopes, and excitements. This moves them from your stewing subconscious onto the objective page in a way that lets them go completely.

Vent to your journal as often as you like, but start by practicing a few times per week. Even when you don't think you have anything to say, write on your set schedule anyway. The items below the surface will come out as you write, and you never would have said them if you hadn't started in the first place.

Sleep Controls Weight

Here's some radical weight control advice—get a good night's sleep.

This is a habit no one really thinks about in regard to their weight and health, but it's a critical part of any lifestyle approach to weight loss. Quality sleep is essential for sustaining the body's normal ability to process and control weight-related functions such as blood sugar levels, cortisol, and thyroid hormones.

The Columbia University Obesity Research Center recently showed that those who got less than four hours of sleep were a full 50 percent more likely to be obese than those getting a normal night of sleep. Dr. Stephen Heymsfield worked on the study and pointed out that "there's growing scientific evidence that there's a link between sleep and the various neural pathways that regulate food intake."

For example, sleep deprivation can manifest itself as hunger cravings, possibly because the hunger hormone grehlin is elevated in the sleep-deprived. For whatever reason, it tends to lead to bingeing and snacking throughout the day. But here's the good news—you don't have to lose sleep over losing sleep. The effects of deprivation can be reversed by just three consecutive full nights of sleep.

Remember that everyone has their own sleep requirements. So I can't make a one-size-fits-all rule to say you absolutely need six hours, eight hours, or ten hours. Everyone has their own physiological needs, and you should get your own normal amount. How do you know what that is? When you wake up refreshed and don't go through the day fatigued, you've got it right.

How do you do that? Below are some simple ways to help your body settle into a comfortable sleep, night after night.

1. *Regular sleep.* To encourage your body to sleep well over the long term, develop a predictable schedule for sleeping, even on weekends. This trains your body to expect to sleep at approximately the same time every night, and wake up at about the same time every morning (whenever possible).

2. *Interrupted sleep.* If you can't sleep one night and decide to get up and do something, be sure that your activity is done in a dimly lit room. Light stimulation can prolong your wakefulness and keep you from going back to sleep.

3. *Alcohol, exercise, and sleep.* It's odd, but alcohol and exercise immediately before bedtime are not sleep aids. Yes, alcohol is chemically a depressant, but it has the effect of decreasing your REM sleep. That's the deep sleep your body must have to feel refreshed in the morning. Exercise makes your body tired but revs up your metabolism and sharpens your mental activity. In fact, exercise right before bed can make it much harder to get to sleep. So if you have a nightcap, make it small. And if you exercise, do it at least two hours before you're ready to go to sleep.

Don't Forget, Don't Diet

Your miraculous body is its own ecosystem of moving parts: genes, cells, tissues, organs, organ systems, emotions, and intellect. All these overlapping elements do their individual jobs, but are linked together to make the entire body function well. The single parts cannot function outside of the context of the whole.

This basic biological reality must be remembered in regard to your weight as well. Thus, any approach to health must embrace the cooperative nature of all the moving parts of the body, not just one or two, or any effects you do see will be short-lived at best. This is precisely why we've found over the past thirty-five years that standard diet strategies fail 90 percent of the time.

The diet mentality is one-dimensional, and therefore unrealistic because it focuses on a single aspect of your body's billion moving parts (accounting for food parts such as carbs, fats, or calories). But sleep affects your weight, stress affects your weight, and your emotional state does, too! You cannot live in this world without the help of those around you, and you cannot live a healthy life without taking care of yourself as a whole person. All these factors conspire as a synergistic unit, and none should be managed outside of the context of the whole.

So sleep well and laugh well. These are the pillars on which you'll build your health. And healthy weight loss will follow as a result.

CHEAT SHEET: FINDING YOUR PEACE

Chronic stress introduces sugar instabilities and weight gain, in addition to the problems it causes for your blood pressure and your heart. Stress reduction comes through laughter, relaxation of body and mind, and a light playful spirit, and there are very simple breathing routines that can help you find your peace every day.

To live a healthy life every day, practice:
- Getting rid of bodily tensions by taking your daily muscle inventory.
- Getting rid of mental tensions by practicing your belly breathing.
- Getting rid of emotional tensions by daily meditation.

The Results You're Looking For

IMMEDIATELY
- Your spirit will feel lighter.
- You will find your thinking clearer.
- You will be more at peace throughout the day.

WITHIN TWO WEEKS
- You will find it easier to laugh, and others will find it easy to laugh around you.
- You will be able to apply your breathing exercises and meditations anytime, anywhere.

WITHIN A MONTH
- You will have made your belly breathing relaxation techniques a natural part of your life.
- Your stress-induced eating episodes will diminish.

HOMEWORK: FOR REDUCING STRESS

1. Do your morning meditation for fifteen minutes, at least three times per week.
2. Practice your belly breathing whenever you feel stressed.
3. Laugh out loud every day.
4. Surround yourself with enjoyable people.
5. Sleep well.

Step ✤ 10

You Don't Have to Go to the Gym

Lyon is France's second largest city—sort of like the Chicago of France. And it offers everything that any other major metropolitan city offers . . . almost.

When I first arrived, my knee was injured and I couldn't even run a mile without it hurting. I'd tried everything, but I had been forced to do other things such as riding stationary bikes or lifting weights. Over lunch, I asked one of the research professors who lived in the Lyon area about the local health clubs.

He stared back at me, processing the request. "Ahh, yes. You mean, like for the mineral bath or spa?"

"No," I said, "like with weight machines, circuit training, sweaty people doing step aerobics," I motioned with my arms. He wasn't getting it. "You know, the banks of stationary bikes, elliptical trainers, rowing machines, free weights, a swimming pool . . ."

"We have swimming pools," he interrupted, a little excited to have found a point of recognition somewhere in my torrent. I asked if he knew anyone who "worked out" there, but he just shook his head.

I ended up blowing off the gym because it was just too hard to communicate the idea. I came to find that they do in fact have their own types of workout facilities in Lyon, but they're remarkably few. For example, if you looked for fitness centers in the Chicago area you'd have a whopping fourteen hundred choices—they're everywhere! A similar search on the official Lyon Web site revealed that there are *no* gyms in that city. Another try returned four options (a mineral bath spa, a pool, some squash courts, and a skateboard arena). In fact, there are a rare few health clubs, but the majority are found in association with hotels (for tourists).

This confirms what I'd seen as well—that the French just don't work out like crazy. According to the International Health, Racquet & Sportsclub Association (IHRSA), the total health club attendees in the United States rose 154 percent from 1987 to 2000, and more than doubled, to 33.8 million, by 2002. Contrast this with the listing for the very largest health club in France, Club Med Gym, which ended the same year with a loss of 62 millions Euros, which followed a loss of 70 million from the year before. This, according to the IHRSA, is why they were recently forced to sell up to seventy-five of their gyms.

In general, we exercise. They don't.

This drives home yet another French paradox. Since science shows that activity really is important for low weight and optimal health, how can we explain the French loathing for sweaty, muscle-aching exercise, when they're so healthy? The answer rests in a distinction we need to understand better—the big difference between exercise and activity. The French are very active, but are not driven to exercise. By contrast, we've heard over and over that you have to practically kill yourself on a workout machine to achieve any effect whatsoever for your health.

The "no pain, no gain" mentality—that you must spend your free time working out at the gym, several times a week, and feel guilty when you don't—is a foreign concept to these thin French people. After all, they would reason, what kind of person seeks out aching muscles?

While we tend to hit the gym, for the most part the French spend their energy walking around. That's it. And they walk because they enjoy it: going to the store, getting outside after dinner, shopping. No one has to bench press or work the rowing machine. Life is not about the sacrifice of having to work through pain at every turn. Life is about seizing the day, about finding the joy and pleasure that sits right there in front of you. The French national sport is hanging out and people watching (and watching the people watchers).

Don't get me wrong, this last step is not about being a couch potato. To lose weight, you really must be active on a daily basis. You just don't have to kill yourself doing it or, worse, feel guilty about not wanting to spend a sunny Saturday slaving away at the gym! In fact, we can even be active when sitting down. Dr. James Levine at the Mayo Clinic in Minnesota found that people who tend to fidget burn up to one hundred more calories per hour than nonfidgeters. This is known as nonexercise activity thermogenesis (NEAT), and simply means that you're being active without exercising.

Doesn't this sound just like every other piece of the French puzzle? You do need water, but you don't need to drown in it. You do need fats and carbs and proteins, but you don't need to overconsume—or cut out completely—any one of them. You do need to be active, but you don't have to exercise.

How the French Stay Active: First Steps to Fitness

Although they don't work out, the French do walk. And when you read this, it sounds so ordinary—everyone does it all the time. But that's actually the best part about it. You can walk anytime, anywhere—and you should. Creatively fill in the spaces of your day with walking activities at every opportunity.

Before you get started on any long hikes, though, be sure to get comfortable shoes and a reasonable pedometer, so you can keep your feet from chafing and keep track of how far you go each day. Many people like to listen to music or other motivational CDs as they walk, and below are more sample situations in which you can step your way to fitness.

Talking

When you're on the phone, cordless technology allows you to walk and talk at the same time. If you have something to share with a friend, or even some issues to work out with someone, take a stroll around the block together. These may be times to walk slowly, but that activity still counts!

Waiting

The elevator won't come, your flight has been delayed, the water on the stove is slow to boil, your meeting has been postponed by thirty minutes, or the kids are in music lessons. When these delays happen, make it your practice to move. You don't have to break a sweat, just move. Walk through the house, around the block, up the stairs. Do it because you can.

Eating

Of course you shouldn't walk while you eat, but you should talk a walk after dinner when you can. It's pleasant, but remember that this is not about working anything off. It's counterproductive to your digestion to do this. This is a peaceful walk, or a grateful stroll of reflection. If this seems odd to you, that's because you're still thinking only in terms of "calories-in, calories-out." That's a very important place to start, but the French lifestyle takes you beyond that limited way of thinking.

Walk to lunch or dinner if you're able to. There's no sense sitting in a car when you could be moving your legs, getting steps in, and enjoying the day.

Working

Even if you work on the one hundredth floor of a skyscraper, walk up the first few flights of stairs and try this experiment. The first time, note how many floors it takes you to get winded. Then see how that number changes over the next week, or two weeks, and track your progress. Every time you extend the number of flights you can ascend, you're boosting your heart health, priming your metabolic rate to burn more calories over a longer period of time, and losing weight in the process!

When you park in the lot, always park on the outside and walk in.

Just be sure to dress well in chilly weather. Remember what the Norwegians say, "There is no bad weather, only bad clothing."

Vacationing
Go hiking and camping whenever you can on vacation. Bring a walking stick and comfortable hiking shoes. If you are traveling in the car, always plan for an extended lunch so you can go for a stroll or play a game afterward.

Free Yourself from the Gym
Simply add an activity you love to your life, and do that instead of going to the gym.

Walk with your friends, bicycle with your kids, go camping with your honey, or garden all by yourself. Although we don't think of them as such, these activities all burn calories and count toward your fitness goals. Engaging in an activity you love every day in lieu of working out at the gym or at home has another wonderful benefit. It prevents you from buying those expensive workout machines that you'll use five days for exercise, and five years for a coat rack.

How to Make the French Approach Work for You: Do What You Love

The French are active, but most don't exercise. This key distinction needs to be remembered if we're ever going to step into a life of fitness. So if you want their fitness success, too, you first must dissect from your mind any notion that you have to suffer to achieve success. You don't!

In fact, the very idea of grunting and straining is enough to keep many people from ever exercising to begin with. And if you do start something you feel like you have to do, you'll either start, stop, and then feel like a failure because you couldn't keep up, or you'll push yourself too hard and injure yourself. Then you'll have to stop anyway!

So just save yourself the pain, and a thousand dollars, and don't even start unless it's something that seems so fun you're absolutely compelled to give it a whirl. And if you want to exercise like the French, then don't exercise . . . be active. Here are just a few ideas, but you should be creative and add your own, as you like.

Dance

When you dance, you burn calories, you laugh (or cry if you have two left feet, like I do), you spend time with friends, and you improve coordination. This is an activity that you'll want to do over and over because it's fun and enjoyable, not because you have to log some hours and monitor your heart rate. Let go, go dance.

Get a Bike and Ride

If you're young you might still want one of those bum-busting seats. But otherwise, get one of the comfortable wide-load, padded, spring-cushioned varieties. Remember, it doesn't have to hurt! Most cities have bike trails on which you can cruise along to feel the breeze brush your hair and clothes. Pack a picnic with your riding partner and stop on some grassy patch for a leisurely bite before heading off again. Bike riding is fabulous for your heart (physically and spiritually) and you'll want to do it over and over.

Pick Your Food

Especially during the summer months, get into the blueberry bushes and strawberry patches and spend the afternoon plucking and picking better produce than you could find anywhere else. And you'll spend less than you will for anything you can find in the store. The acts of bending and reaching and walking and squatting and standing (and nibbling!) burn calories in a healthy way. Think of it as the perfect combination of nutrition and fitness.

Window Shop

This is a great activity, especially with someone who shares your fetish for bargain grazing. You can drop your cruising velocity when you close in on your favorite stores, but pick up your pace between them to get to as many sales as possible. And when you have to go up a level, never take the escalators or elevators unless you absolutely have to.

Practice Yoga

Yoga is the perfect exercise for the chronic multitasker (even the word *yoga* means *union* in the ancient Indian language of Sanskrit, where yoga originated). Most people think of yoga as simply stretching, but in practice it also strengthens your muscles and relaxes your mind. So if you're interested in one-stop shopping for stress relief, stretching, and muscle toning, yoga is a perfect exercise.

And the other very good reason multitaskers will love yoga is precisely because of its stress-reducing benefits. You can practice yoga with a group, if you need the structure of meeting times, but it's very easy to do in your own home as well, at your convenience. You don't need special equipment—just a floor, perhaps a yoga mat, and a few minutes of your day.

Play Games

Try tennis, soccer, badminton, bowling . . . it doesn't matter. Just enroll yourself in something you can love and do consistently. Many of these kinds of games have a season or structure, so you can do it for a while before moving on to something else.

A dear friend of mine is an enthusiastic Ping-Pong player. Often when we visit, Adam and I will hang around politely until the moment we can sneak away and have a cutthroat, Australian rules, no-holds-barred "tournament." We have great fun for an hour or so of batting a little ball around a table. This is a perfect fitness routine.

Remember that the point of these activities is fun and enjoyment. The effect is fitness. Thus, don't make the mistake of thinking you have to be good at any of these games. You don't have to be Tiger Woods to swing a golf club and have a good time. The point is the play.

No, these activities won't require that you hyperanalyze your heart rate as generally recommended by some fitness experts—calculate your maximum rate (220 − your age × 70 percent) to get your target rate and then take 85 percent of that number as the number of heartbeats to maintain for twenty minutes on average . . . whew! Who's going to do that for long, except people so fanatically into fitness that they don't have weight problems anyway! Being so agenda-oriented is the fitness equivalent of asking someone to diet by micromanaging carbs, fats, proteins, and calories throughout every day. You may crunch the numbers once or twice, but then you get tired of it, can't continue, and feel defeated.

The good news? It turns out that an overeager approach to exercise isn't even necessary for weight loss. New studies reveal that short bouts of activity spread throughout the day are just as effective at improving your aerobic fitness. Even walking for ten minutes three times during the day, according to a recent study by Drs. Murphy and Hardman, is just as good for your fitness level as one thirty-minute walking workout. Much of this new research on the "slow exercise" movement—analogous to the Italian "slow food" movement—has been done by Glenn Gaesser, an exercise physiologist at the University of Virginia. He advises that people must "get out of the all-or-nothing mind-set that, unless they exercise for 30 minutes, they're wasting their time."

The Irony of Convenience

Taking the time out of your day to enjoy your life doesn't encourage sloth any more than loving your food has anything to do with gluttony. It's about engaging in the world around you. That may mean walking when you could drive, taking the stairs instead of elevators, or playing with your kids instead of watching from a distance. In fact, sometimes convenience and labor-saving devices are exactly what stand between us and lifelong fitness.

Try this thought experiment by taking the notion of convenience to its logical extreme. At some point, can conveniences become a bad thing? At some point, do labor-saving tools become harmful, instead of helpful?

Imagine what it was like when people had to tote their own laundry down to a stream about a mile from their home. They might spend all day just doing laundry. Thank goodness that indoor plumbing and the washer and dryer came along. These really helped. With electricity and gas, we don't have to chop wood to cook food. What a wonderful benefit. And, with each new invention over the past one hundred years, we've progressed along this path that continually maximizes leisure and minimizes movement.

But how much convenience is enough? What if someone did your work for you, mowed your yard, drove you around, and even set you in a rolling chair so you could move at the slightest push of a button, and you wouldn't have to walk for yourself? What a convenience—or is it? Do you know anyone who does this? Most likely, you're picturing someone who's disabled. These are people who would give anything they had for the luxury of inconvenience: to walk, take the stairs by themselves, or go to the store on their own.

There is a line over which convenience becomes debilitation, and the search for labor-saving devices becomes sloth. The question is, where is that line?

There's nothing wrong with timesaving efforts, but as we've seen over and over, anything taken to an extreme becomes extremely unhealthy for you. Bear this in mind when you have the opportunity to walk a few more feet or to get outside on the weekend: being active is not a liability but a gift you would ache for as soon as you had to be pushed around in a wheelchair or have someone do your shopping or tend your garden for you.

So nurture your gifts. If you spend your life trying to find ways to avoid walking, standing, and just moving, your wish may be granted. To avoid this fate, move every chance you get: up the stairs, from the far end of the parking lot, when you're on break, when you're on the phone.

Daily Activities That Really Do Burn Calories

- Lawn mowing: burns up to 400 calories per hour.
- Gardening: burns up to 400 calories per hour.
- Strolling while talking on your cell phone: burns 300 calories per hour.
- Doing light housework while watching TV: burns 200 calories per hour.
- Typing: burns 113 calories per hour.
- Standing: burns 140 calories per hour.
- Raking leaves: burns 225 calories per hour.
- Throwing a Frisbee in your free time: burns 225 calories per hour.
- Having sex: burns 190 calories per hour (your individual mileage may vary).
- Taking the stairs instead of the elevator: burns 100 calories per day.

⚜ *Problem: I don't have enough energy to be active.*

You hear this all the time: "I eat a lot because I have a big appetite."

You also hear this: "I'm too tired to go out and exercise."

Both of these statements should be reversed. You have a big appetite *because you eat so much.* We talked a great deal in Step 4 about how you can train your body to expect larger quantities of food, just by your behavioral habits. But the same is true for your activity levels. People can become sluggish, in part, *because they don't move.*

The worst part of this is that you can get into a negative circle of inactivity, which makes you lethargic, which makes you inactive, which makes you lethargic, and on and on. At this point, you're circling the drain.

Solution: Be intentional.

The way out of this downward spiral is to be active *on purpose,* which will increase your ability to be active by boosting your overall energy in the long term. Why is that?

Have you ever exercised right before bed? When you do, you find that it's hard to fall right to sleep because you're heart is still pounding and your metabolism is way up. The elevated metabolic rate is a temporary phenomenon that becomes permanent when you're consistent. And, when your body's metabolism is cranked up, you have more energy. This becomes a positive feedback loop that supports even more activity!

So, to shake yourself out of the lethargic blahs that keep you from being active . . . go out there and *be* active! Manually kick-start your metabolic engine, to train your body to boost your energy level and burn calories throughout the day. It's okay to start with small additions to your daily activity, but you must add something. You can add longer periods of activity later, as it makes sense to you.

⚜ PEOPLE ON THE PATH

Dear Will,

When I was a child, I was as skinny as could be. I ate what I wanted when I wanted to. It was great. Unfortunately, however, I grew up and started gaining weight in my twenties and more in my thirties and forties. When I started dieting in my thirties, the roller coaster began. I'd lose fifteen pounds and gain twenty pounds. I hated the way I looked and I hated the fact that I could no longer eat the things I loved. I tried all the no-fat foods out there thinking they would help, but they didn't and I still hated my food.

I was so excited when I saw your eating plan—it made immediate sense to me. Faux foods were out the door immediately. My twenty-one-year-old daughter and I cleaned out the refrigerator, freezer, and cupboards. We rid ourselves of every item that had high-fructose corn syrup in it or ingredients that we didn't recognize as real food. That was easy and fun. We went grocery shopping and stuck with fresh foods. Fruits and vegetables, meat, chicken and fish, and bread. Oh, how I love bread. We started lingering longer over our meals. Enjoying every bite. Savoring each flavor.

Next, the accomplishment that I am the proudest about: I stopped drinking diet soda. I have been a soda-holic my whole life and I easily stopped drinking it. I haven't had a soda in almost three months. It took me close to fifty years to start eating the right way and I can't begin to tell you how great I feel.

I just bought myself a pedometer and challenge myself to walk five miles a day. I keep track of how many steps I walk in a daily journal. My family and I are really enjoying this approach to healthy living. Mealtime has become a special occasion every night thanks to you.

—Jean L.

How Can I Increase My Metabolism Without Going to the Gym?

As we've said, being active is like putting money in the metabolic bank, because it revs up your metabolism—a word that simply reflects the amount of energy your body needs for all its organs and tissues. With a higher resting metabolism, your body uses up more energy while you're not exercising, even while you're sleeping. In fact, this basic energy demand is believed to account for around 70 percent of your total daily calorie expenditure.

In fact, your resting metabolism is one of the chief reasons standard diets of calorie restriction do not work—because they lower your metabolic rate! So you may be eating less, but you're burning less as well. When you return to normal eating patterns, with that depressed metabolism, any weight you did lose comes right back.

One very important key to cranking up your metabolic rate is to increase your muscle tone. You don't have to bulk up (have you ever seen a muscle-bound Frenchman?), but being active builds lean muscles, which burn more energy even when they don't happening to be flexing. Each pound of lean muscle burns about thirty-five calories per day. Thus, going for muscle tone is the metabolic equivalent of learning healthy eating habits. Once you have them, their benefits continue to silently work for you in the background—so you don't have to think about them all the time.

Activities to Tone Your Muscles

If you want to adopt a reasonable balance between the French laissez-faire approach to exercise and the gung-ho approach, a wonderful middle ground can be the series of simple toning activities we list here. And only ten minutes of low-level tone building per day is all you need to make this happen. Choose any of the simple movements below, and make just ten minutes for yourself at some time during the day—mornings are best. You'll start to see concrete results, such as weight loss, in the first two weeks. The only caveat is to work different muscles on different days so you don't overtax any single muscle group.

Here are the general rules. Repeat each exercise ten times, or until fatigued. Hold each posture for one full second during each repetition. Do each set of ten movements three times. If you get tired, don't worry. Expect to increase the number of repetitions your body can do as you continue.

Legs

FOR YOUR HAMSTRINGS: Lie on your back on the floor with your feet (flat) up on the seat of a chair in front of you and your legs slightly bent. Press down with your feet on the chair to extend your legs and arch your back. Hold for one full second in this arched position. Return to the original position.

FOR YOUR QUADRICEPS: Stand in front of a chair, facing away from it, and *slowly* sit down to lightly touch the seat. Be sure to keep your back straight. Hold. Return to standing.

FOR YOUR CALVES: Stand on a stair (at the bottom of a flight) with your heels extended over the edge and only the balls of your feet on the step. Allow your heels to drop as far down as they will go. Then slowly rise onto your toes. Hold. Return.

FOR YOUR INNER AND OUTER THIGHS: Lie on your side with your legs slightly apart so that you can raise your lower leg. While the upper leg remains still, lift the lower leg slowly up as far as you can. Hold. Slowly return to floor. Next, lift your top leg up slowly as far as you can. Hold. Return. When you've completed each leg, switch to the other side.

FOR YOUR BUM: From a position on your hands and knees, slowly extend your right leg straight back as far *out and up* as you can. Hold that posture for a long count of one. Slowly return to the starting position. Repeat with your left leg. You'll probably need to be on a mat or something soft, so you don't hurt your knees.

Arms

FOR YOUR SHOULDERS: Weights can be used, but they aren't necessary if you don't have them. Sit in a chair with your hands extended to your knees. And, if you like, hold light weights (or something that weighs about five pounds) in each hand. Keeping your arms extended, slowly raise your hands to the level of your head. Hold. Repeat. (See A Note About Weights, page 237.)

FOR YOUR CHEST: Do a simple push-up either from your knees or from your toes. Be sure to keep your back straight (do not bend at the waist). Slowly bend your arms until your body touches the floor. Hold. Return.

FOR YOUR BICEPS: Sit in a comfortable chair and grab a weight of between two to ten pounds, depending on what you can lift easily. Begin with your arm extended and your elbow placed on your thigh. Slowly curl the weight up toward your shoulder until your arm is completely flexed. Hold in that position for a long count of one. Return to the extended position.

FOR YOUR TRICEPS: Find any fixed object in your house (for example, bathtub or cabinet countertop). Facing away from it, put your hands behind you on the edge. Make sure you have a good grip and then step your feet in front of you until your weight is resting on your hands. Keep your legs straight, and slowly bend your arms until they are roughly at a 90-degree angle. Hold. Return to the arms-extended position. You will find that the higher the object is that you are grasping, the easier this exercise will be.

A Note About Weights

The point of these exercises is not to build muscle bulk, but to tone muscle, increase your resting metabolic rate, and therefore remove fat. To do this, keep in mind that you need to choose a weight that feels too light to begin with. But, because you're doing each exercise ten times, it will certainly feel heavier as you go. So start with a very light weight and do these exercises for a week or so. If you experience soreness, back off on the weight or the number of reps. If it hurts, don't do it.

Axis Muscles

FOR YOUR LOWER ABDOMINALS: Try simple leg raises. Lie on the floor on your back, bend one leg to support you and extend the other. Slowly lift the extended leg about twelve inches off the ground. Hold. Return slowly to the ground.

FOR YOUR UPPER ABDOMINALS: Lie on your back with your feet up and your knees bent at 90 degrees. With your hands across your chest, curl your shoulders upward so they are about three inches off the floor. Hold. Slowly return.

FOR YOUR LOWER BACK: Lie on your stomach with your hands extended in front of you. Slowly arch your torso and legs off the ground in the shape of a bow. Hold. Return slowly to floor.

These activities take very little time, are easy to do, and burn energy for you without your ever having to think about them. And all you have to commit to is ten minutes per day. The key here is to be consistent and to mix muscle groups from one day to another. Here's a sample routine that works wonders: leg movements one day, arms the next, axis muscles on the third day, take a break on day four, and then repeat. Simple!

What If I Love to Work Out?

I've said that you don't have to go to the gym, and also that you don't have to exercise. But that doesn't mean you must avoid it altogether if you love that sort of thing. Personally, I do. My family and I take karate, and it's a blast to get out there and scream in the air, kick in the air, punch in the air. I learn something new about this art every time I go, and let me tell you it's a sweaty workout.

But the point is that I love it. It's not something I feel compelled to do just because of some arbitrary idea about the requirements for being fit.

If jogging in place on a treadmill is something you couldn't do without, please don't give it up. If oscillating on a stair stepper for thirty minutes lights you up, by all means continue to do it. Just do it because you love it, not because you feel guilty. This way you'll never trudge through two weeks of some workout regime that you completely dislike.

Don't Forget, Don't Diet

How do you know that our French approach is a "way of life" and not just another quick-fix fad diet? Because it applies general principles that work wonderfully across the board: in your food choices, eating routines, methods for stress management, and even fitness. It allows you to stop straining so hard to see what's right in front of you, to let go, and to embrace your own *joie de vivre*.

Physical fitness fits perfectly into the very same theme. Follow your heart and do what you love every day. Yes, be active, but don't think you have to put yourself through overt pain and suffering to achieve lifelong effects—this is something we've been told, but it just isn't true. The thin, healthy people of the world outlive the rest of us, have less risk of heart disease, and a lower obesity rate without our type A fitness fanaticism—and they're relaxed using this approach.

So your task is to find activities you can love to do every day. If laughing and friends and conversation are involved somehow, so much the better! This general guideline frees you workout-a-holics up to go pound the treadmill or pump iron if you like. But it also releases the rest of us from the belief that you *have to do that* to be fit and healthy. It opens your fitness goals to enjoyment and, in the end, you'll move more every day, enjoy the process, and stick with it longer.

The result? A longer, fitter, happier life.

CHEAT SHEET: MOVIN' & GROOVIN'

Be active, even if you don't exercise. Fill your life with movements you love to do, instead of painfully boring routines you feel like you have to do. That way you'll stick with it longer, have more fun doing it, and get more fit in the process!

Get Moving
- Find an activity or two you love to do, and get engaged.
- Give up the onerous exercises designed to "whip you into shape."
- Make your exercise social whenever you can.
- Tone your muscles to increase your metabolism.
- Walk, every chance you get.

The Results You're Looking For

IMMEDIATELY
- You will add pleasure to your fitness approach.
- You will add activities that don't even feel like exercise.

WITHIN TWO WEEKS
- Your cardiovascular system will respond with greater efficiency and a longer time before reaching exhaustion.
- Your toned muscles will be working for you even when you sleep. This is when you'll notice that your clothes are fitting better!

WITHIN A MONTH

- Your walking routines will become such a normal part of your life that you won't have to think about them.
- At this point, you'll be living an active life for good.

HOMEWORK: ACTIVITY

1. Unless you absolutely love it, give up painful types of exercise.
2. Take up some activity that excites you, makes you laugh, or gives you happiness.
3. Add toning activities for the first two weeks, alternating muscle groups on different days. If you are comfortable with them after this time period, continue.
4. Be creative about adding walking into your day. Every chance you get, walk.

Real Meal Plans

A ren't standard diet book meal plans hopeless? They tell you to eat specific foods on specific days and at specific times, with some stunning new creation every day. The following breakfast meal plan actually came straight out of one popular diet book. I want to imagine yourself actually doing this for even one week.

> **Mon:** Peach quick bread, fresh raspberries; **Tue:** Blueberry muffin with lemon glaze, cantaloupe wedge; **Wed:** Yogurt layered with granola, fruit, and coconut; **Thurs:** Cereal bar, yogurt topped with blueberries; **Fri:** Mini-bagel with jam and reduced-fat cream cheese, yogurt with sliced peach; **Sat:** Vegetable frittata wedge, wheat toast, blueberries; **Sun:** Pancakes with light syrup, sliced strawberries.

And this was just breakfast! It sounds great in theory, but no one with a life can do it, which makes the point perfectly: overmanaging your schedule and expectations sets you up for one big dietary downfall.

So the meal plan we've designed is a flexible template that you can adapt as necessary in your busy life. We include example foods for breakfast, lunch, and dinner that you can add as you like. Eat yogurt and fruit, or a bagel with cream cheese, every morning if that's what you love. Remember, the French approach is about principles for living, not dietary dictation.

The meal plan goes beyond just the food. To live a healthy lifestyle, you have to incorporate the habits of healthy eating as well. With each meal and each day, you'll find tips to make your new approach work in the real world. With *what to eat* and *how to eat* covered in this user-friendly framework, these meal plans become practical, useful, and tasty.

Breakfast (Target time: 15 to 20 minutes)

Select any whole grain, balanced lightly with a little butter, peanut butter, or cream cheese. There really is no ender for breakfast, unless you save your coffee until after the meal.

Alternatively, select yogurt with any fresh or dried fruit. Your drink in these cases can be 100 percent fruit juice, milk, water, coffee, or tea. However, fruit juice will not be as good for you as the fruit itself—an orange is better than orange juice, an apple is better than apple juice.

Eggs are perfect foods, when limited to one or two per day, prepared to your liking. If you fry them, extra-virgin olive or vegetable oil can be used as well as butter.

Oats are healthful for the heart, take ten minutes to make, and the added goodness of fiber is a bonus that goes perfectly with a pat of butter, a little brown sugar, and a good solid sprinkle of cinnamon.

Breakfast main _____
Drink _____

LIFESTYLE TIP OF THE MEAL: Wake up thirty minutes early. Sit in the peace of your kitchen to begin your day with your partner, paper, or your favorite cup of coffee.

If you eat at home and want to cook, try having

> One egg prepared to your liking.
> One portion of some grain, such as whole-wheat bread, grits, oats, or half a bagel.

LIFESTYLE TIP OF THE MEAL: Practice this habit until it becomes automatic. Wait a minute or two after all the food is completely out of your mouth before picking up your food again.

If you're in a hurry, try having

> Two-thirds bowl of oatmeal (see the recipe for Brown Sugar Cinnamon Oatmeal, page 272) or the yogurt/granola/fruit combination.

LIFESTYLE TIP OF THE MEAL: Make your meal about more than just mindless consumption. Take a breather between bites from time to time to chat or read or do something else. You'll enjoy your food more when you do come back to it.

If you have to eat on the road, try having

> Breakfast at a local diner with real foods such as eggs, potatoes, and so on. You can also find restaurants that serve freshly made bagels and cream cheese.

LIFESTYLE TIP OF THE MEAL: If you're traveling by yourself, bring a good book so you won't have to eat alone.

Lunch (Target time: 20 to 30 minutes)

Select any series of main and side dishes from the lunch suggestions that follow.

Lunch main _____

Side(s) _____   _____

Drinks _____

Dessert or ender _____

Lunches are typically the same size or a bit smaller than dinners. When you eat out, you might have a soup and half sandwich (or just one of those) with a salad and buttered bread—just make sure the bread is real. Alternatively, many people just bring leftovers in to work from home.

Some work conditions may make it difficult to separate the meal out into courses, so you must focus on your eating habits to prolong the time. Another solution, if you're feeling rushed, is to take your meal back to your desk to finish it there. It's far better to do this than to gobble it down.

If you're eating on the road and stop at a reasonable (non–fast food) restaurant, go ahead and have the standard main, starch, and veggie, as long as you're prepared to box up about half of the food they serve and take it back with you. Don't eat their fried foods, because they will have been made in a vat of oils. Baked and grilled are better. Other than that, most sit-down restaurants have acceptable real food.

As for your dessert and ender, remember that if you have a rich dessert you shouldn't also have a rich ender. For example, if you have no dessert, then a creamy bit of cheese for the ender is perfect (the size of four dice, no more). But following a luscious rich dessert, coffee and tea are perfect enders that help carry you through the early afternoon. Just make sure to sip it and make it last.

LIFESTYLE TIP OF THE MEAL: Estimate the size of half of your sandwich before you begin, and resolve to finish with that half only after seven to ten minutes or so.

If you're at a restaurant, try having

Coleslaw as your side instead of fries
Or a salad with grilled salmon or chicken
A la carte soup, fresh bread, and a side only

LIFESTYLE TIP OF THE MEAL: Salad dressing complements the flavors of the salad—but many people load too much of it on, resulting in a huge source of needless calories. Put just enough dressing on your salad to enhance the flavor, no more.

If you're in a hurry, try having

Any of your leftovers—serve them from your container onto your plate, and then put away the food so you don't overconsume.
Bread dipped in olive oil, tomato with mozzarella cheese and basil.
Sardines or kippers on a good cracker, baby carrots dipped in an all natural dip (such as hummus).
A wonderful dessert to try is any cut fruit with a splash of cream.

LIFESTYLE TIP OF THE MEAL: Never eat on your feet, at the sink, or by the stove. Always sit down and give your meal the attention it deserves. Enjoyment of the meal is more about the time spent than the amount eaten.

If you take your lunch to work, try having

A single sandwich on healthful bread with light veggies on the side, such as sliced red bell peppers. Normally, you don't need bread on both sides of your sandwich—just eat it open-faced.
A leftover main course, such as a grilled chicken breast, is fabulous served with a dip of mixed mayonnaise and horseradish sauce, or spicy mustard and roasted garlic.

Soup supplemented with fresh bread from the cafeteria or nearby bakery.

LIFESTYLE TIP OF THE MEAL: Don't let the size of your food determine the size of your bite. Cut your pieces into reasonably small bites on purpose.

Dinner (Target time: 30 minutes or longer)

The rule for dinner is the same as the rule for lunch. Always include a balance of foods such as protein, veggies, and starches. Remember that you cannot have dessert unless you've saved room for it by eating small along the way.

Select any series of main and side dishes from the dinner suggestions that follow.

Dinner main _____

Side(s) _____   _____

Drinks _____

Dessert or ender _____

Dinners will vary depending on whether you have a snacky dinner, leftovers, a home-cooked meal, or go out to a restaurant. No matter which you choose, always take enough time to enjoy yourself. Sit and talk and relax.

LIFESTYLE TIP OF THE MEAL: Turn off all technology except the answering machine during the meal.

If you're in a hurry, try having

Fish broiled for 20 minutes with olive oil, garlic salt, lemon pepper, and thyme.

Orzo pasta with Parmesan, pine nuts, and chopped sun-dried tomatoes.

A spinach salad with chopped tomatoes and walnuts.

A salad dressing of olive oil, balsamic vinegar, oregano, salt and pepper, and a touch of Dijon mustard.

Avgolemono soup: heat chicken stock with a handful of rice and leftover shredded chicken until the rice is done; slowly drizzle one cup of the hot soup into a mixture of one egg and the juice from one lemon; slowly add that back to the main pot and you're ready.

Toasted bread, buttered and rubbed with a cut garlic clove.

LIFESTYLE TIP OF THE MEAL: To prevent rushing through a meal, focus on calming activities just before it starts.

If you order takeout, try having chinese food with no MSG, pizza at places where the ingredients are freshly prepared, or Mexican where you know the tortillas are not made with hydrogenated oils. Just be sure to serve your food from the cartons onto your plates. For example, don't set the delivery box in your lap or that becomes one big portion for you.

LIFESTYLE TIP OF THE MEAL: You know when you order to-go boxes that you'll get more than you need. So practice the habit of always leaving a little bit of food on your plate at the end of your meal, and put the rest away. Even leftover night can be fun. Set the table. Chill the wine. Set out the candles.

Breakfast Suggestions

If you can cook on that day:

Oats (see Brown Sugar Cinnamon Oatmeal, page 272)
Egg cooked to your liking

Scones

Biscuits (see Somebody's Buttermilk Biscuits, page 300)

Pancakes (see Banana Nut Pancakes, page 273)

If you cannot cook on that day:

Bagel with cream cheese or butter (½ bagel is one portion)

Cereal (if sugar is not one of the top 3 ingredients)

A balance of fruit and fat:

Cut fruit with a touch of cream

Peanut butter and any kind of fruit

Granola with yogurt and fruit of your choosing

Cut mango and brie cheese

Lunch and Dinner Suggestions Are the Same

Balance your lunch or dinner with a little protein, starch, and some veggies. The lists of the elements of lunch and dinner are by no means exhaustive, and you can add in your own as you like. Remember, you can eat anything you want, as long as it is real food and you eat small. The only real limitation to this rule involves the kinds of meats you choose. Rely on fish and chicken, have pork when it is lean, and eat red meat very sparingly (twice per month, for example).

PROTEIN

Tarragon Tuna Salad (page 293)

Chicken salad

Any baked fish, such as salmon or Tilapia with Sherry and Rosemary (page 277)

Lean pork roast or chop

Chicken, prepared to your liking (try Red Roasted Chicken, page 281; Chicken Potpie in Sherry Cream Sauce, page 283; and Braised Orange Chicken, page 287)

Three-bean salad

Black bean chili

STARCH

Homemade Baguettes (page 298) or other bread

Macaroni and Cheese (page 307)

Pasta salad

Buttermilk Cornbread (page 306)

Baked baby red potatoes with rosemary

Mashed potatoes with sour cream and butter

Any legumes, such as white beans, red beans, black beans, Baked
Beans (page 301)

Homemade french fries (and try them made with sweet potatoes!)

Steamed rice or Pine Nut Parmesan Risotto (page 310)

Corn on the cob, or as you enjoy it

Biscotti (try Double-Almond Biscotti, page 268)

VEGETABLES

Sliced tomatoes with drizzle of olive oil and balsamic vinegar

Steamed broccoli with a touch of butter and lemon

Broccoli cut small and stir-fried with walnuts

Any tossed salad with any added goodies you like

Sautéed summer squash

Grilled veggie kabobs

Coleslaw (try Cancer-Fighting Coleslaw, page 303)

Red onion baked in red wine and red wine vinegar

Sautéed sliced onions with mushrooms

Sliced tomato and avocado salad with mozzarella

Garlic green beans with a spritz of lemon on top

Artichokes in a garlic mayonnaise dip (try Hot Artichoke-Cheese
Dip, page 257)

Asparagus baked with Parmesan, salt, and pepper

DESSERTS

Brownie with walnuts (try Chewy Chocolate Brownies,
page 314)

Ice cream

Dark chocolate

Any pudding (try Vanilla Pudding, page 325)

Any dessert bread (try Molasses Gingerbread Cake,
page 318)

Chocolate cake (try Practically Flourless Chocolate Cake,
page 316)

Apple pie (try All-American Apple Pie, page 321)

Any fresh fruit

Any red fruit coated in real chocolate ganache (try Magic Chocolate Ganache, page 324)

Fruit cobbler (try Cuppa Cuppa Cuppa Apple Cobbler, page 319)

If you are having a single dish lunch:

Chicken Potpie in Sherry Cream Sauce (page 283)

Soup such as French Onion Soup (page 292)

Salad with protein and veggies included, such as a Cobb salad

Pizza (try Healthful Pepperoni Pizza, page 294)

Quiche, any variety

Pasta in a tomato-based or cream-based sauce

Chili with Cheddar cheese and sour cream

Gumbo with rice

Lasagna, veggie or regular (try The Last Lasagna, page 278)

Burrito or fajita with beans, guacamole, sour cream, and grilled
veggies

Hamburger, if homemade

If you are having a snack:

Hummus, as a dip with baby carrots or spread onto a pita

Fresh bread dipped in olive oil and balsamic vinegar with oregano
and cayenne (or other spices to your taste)

Quick crostini of toast rubbed with garlic, a slice of tomato, sprinkle of feta, touch of olive oil, salt and pepper, and oregano to
season. Then toast again.

Sliced avocado, tomato, and mozzarella with basil, served with
    toast and white wine

Roasted garlic on toast, served with a handful of walnuts and
    eaten with blue cheese

Any red fruit with chocolate that's been melted slowly with a
    touch of cream in it

Tart apple with sharp Cheddar cheese, both thinly sliced

Soft-boiled egg with garlic-rubbed toast

Artichoke leaves with garlic mayonnaise dip

Easy Recipes for Fabulous Foods

The French approach to good health may seem intimidating if you think that you must be a brilliant chef to make good food. In fact, this is the response I got from so many people after publication of *The Fat Fallacy:* "French? I can't cook French! I don't have the hat, I haven't taken cooking courses, and I don't have three hours to destroy my kitchen!"

But as any French mother will tell you, the French do cook at home and it's very easy to do. Yes, a chef may know just how to whip his eggs into restaurant-ready meringue, but you can make fabulous meals with just a few ingredients and in just a few minutes. It's not hard, we're just told it is by the food companies that would rather have you purchase their products than tomatoes, onions, and garlic.

One of the problems we face is that we've become so used to the instant, fake versions of real foods that many people simply don't know how to make them anymore. Do you know how to make buttermilk biscuits? An apple pie? Brownies? If you don't, you'll certainly end up buying the boxed stuff and eating their preservatives, dyes, and trans fats, just because you didn't know how to make the alternatives.

These recipes were designed specifically for you, to replace some of our most common faux foods with real foods. These are all recipes I make at home, and I've included the tips and tricks that I use in my own kitchen. Once you try these a few times, you won't even have to refer to the recipes, and you'll be eating more healthfully than you ever have before.

Bon appétit!

Recipe List by Category

Creamy Alfredo Sauce

This Alfredo sauce is so easy to make that it becomes a perfect "starter recipe" if you are new to cooking. Moreover, you can make it in the time it takes your pasta water to boil.

Time to the Table: 7 minutes ❧ *Makes enough for about 4 servings*

YOU'LL NEED

2 tablespoons unsalted butter

½ cup heavy cream

¾ cup grated Parmesan cheese

Freshly ground black pepper

IN A SAUCEPAN

Over medium-high heat, melt the butter. Then add the cream, Parmesan, and pepper and warm until the cheese is melted. Correct the seasonings, and mix into your pasta.

Play with Your Food!

For a silkier version of the Alfredo sauce, just add eggs. Mix in 2 beaten eggs with the cream off the heat, and then add the warm melted butter to that mixture (beat it in to make sure the eggs warm slowly).

To make a Carbonara, add about 4 pieces of crisp bacon, crumbled, to the sauce.

FAUX-FOOD EQUIVALENT: *Knorr Fettuccine Pasta with Alfredo Sauce*

Ingredients: Enriched noodles, cheese powders (cow's milk, cheese cultures, salt, enzymes, calcium chloride, sodium hexametaphosphate), salt, cream powder (cream, nonfat dry milk, whey, sodium caseinate, soybean oil, lecithin), hydrogenated soybean oil, lactose, modified food starch, monosodium glutamate, autolyzed yeast extract, maltodextrin, whey protein concentrate, buttermilk, butter, disodium phosphate, sodium nitrate, garlic powder, onion powder, whey, corn syrup solids, vinegar powder, spices, mono- and diglycerides, natural flavors.

Tricks of the Trade

Before adding the eggs, make sure the mixture has cooled off enough so the eggs don't curdle in the pan.

If the sauce is too thick, thin it by adding a bit more water, one tablespoon at a time.

Lemonless Béarnaise Sauce

Best for steak, but it also works for chicken and salmon. What you'll notice every time is how much this sauce tastes like lemons—but there's not one lemon in it!

Time to the Table: 7 minutes ❖ *Makes enough for about 4 servings*

YOU'LL NEED

1 tablespoon minced shallots

½ teaspoon dried tarragon

2 tablespoons white wine

2 tablespoons white wine vinegar

3 large egg yolks, beaten with 1 tablespoon water

½ cup (1 stick) unsalted butter, cubed

Salt and pepper to taste

IN A HEAVY-BOTTOMED SAUCEPAN

Simmer the shallots, tarragon, wine, and vinegar until reduced, and you are left with about 2 tablespoons liquid. Set this off the heat and allow to cool.

ASSEMBLE THE SAUCE

Add the beaten egg yolks and water to the cooled tarragon-vinegar reduction. Turn the heat to medium-low. Stirring or whisking constantly, add the butter a few cubes at a time until all are incorporated. Season with salt and pepper to taste and serve warm.

Play with Your Food

This rich sauce is the second cousin of hollandaise. For extra flavor, add Dijon mustard or horseradish (½ teaspoon should do it). For a sweeter twist, especially when serving with salmon, add a tablespoon of orange juice.

FAUX-FOOD EQUIVALENT: *McCormick Béarnaise Sauce Blend*

Ingredients: Nonfat dry milk, wheat starch, salt, onion, autolyzed yeast extract, butter, maltodextrin, spices, chicken broth, hydrolyzed corn gluten, soy protein, wheat gluten, modified corn starch, xanthan gum, garlic, vinegar solids, gelatin, paprika, citric acid, turmeric, natural flavors, sodium caseinate, sugar, extracts of tarragon.

Hot Artichoke-Cheese Dip

You can make batch after batch of this dip as needed, since it takes only a few minutes to mix together. When it comes out of the oven, you'll see why the kitchen is always the most popular room at any good party.

Time to the Table: 35 minutes ❦ Makes enough for about 15 servings

YOU'LL NEED

1 15-ounce can artichokes, drained and chopped

1 cup grated Parmesan cheese

1¼ cups mayonnaise

½ teaspoon garlic salt

2 full turns of a pepper grinder

2 dashes of Tabasco sauce

2 dashes of cayenne pepper

Tricks of the Trade

If you like finding bits of artichokes in your dip, be careful when mixing up these canned artichokes, as they mash very easily.

Preheat the oven to 350°F.

IN AN OVEN-SAFE CASSEROLE DISH

Mix the artichokes, Parmesan, mayonnaise, garlic salt, pepper, Tabasco sauce, and cayenne until basically smooth.

Bake until bubbly, with a hint of brown on the surface (look in on your dip after about 30 minutes).

Play with Your Food

For extra bite, add a third (or fourth) dash of cayenne pepper.

You don't have to use Parmesan; any hard cheese will work in this dip. Asiago is a good one to try for a saltier flavor. Not only can you vary the cheese, but add an extra half cup if you think it needs it. Your company will only thank you.

FAUX-FOOD EQUIVALENT: *Fromage Per Favor Cheese Dip*

Ingredients: Gorgonzola and feta cheese, mayonnaise (soybean oil, egg yolks, salt, sugar, distilled vinegar, salt, lemon juice concentrate [contains sodium bisulfite]), flavoring (partially hydrogenated soybean oil, tert-butylhydroquinone [TBHQ], tocopherols, synthetic mustard oil, fractionated vegetable oil), coloring (paprika, annatto, soybean oil, gum arabic, natural flavor, ascorbic acid), red peppers, olives (olives, water, pimento, salt, lactic acid, sodium alginate, guar gum, calcium chloride), ripe olives (olives, water, salt, ferrous gluconate).

Authentic French Dressing

Our North American version of French dressing is rarely seen in France. There really is a "French Dressing," although our neon-orange attempt is definitely not it. The real thing is incredibly simple to put together, and contains only a handful of ingredients. What it doesn't contain is artificial colors and, as pointed out by Julia Child, sugar in salad dressing "is heresy."

Time to the Table: 5 minutes ✤ *Makes 1 cup*

YOU'LL NEED

¾ *cup extra-virgin olive oil*

¼ *cup red wine vinegar*

Salt, pepper, and/or other seasonings to taste (tarragon is a wonderful addition)

IN A SMALL MIXING BOWL

Whisk together the olive oil, vinegar, and seasonings.

Make this fresh each time, because all you are doing is mixing your oil and vinegar with whatever herbs happen to be fresh in your garden at the time.

Play with Your Food

If you like it spicy, drop in a teaspoon of Dijon mustard or a sprinkle of cayenne pepper.

FAUX-FOOD EQUIVALENT: *Kraft Creamy French Dressing*

Ingredients: Soybean oil, water, sugar, vinegar, salt, whey, paprika, xanthan gum, sorbic acid, calcium disodium ethylenediamine tetra-acetic acid (EDTA), polysorbate 60, dried garlic, propylene glycol alginate, Yellow No. 6, Yellow No. 5, natural flavor.

A Mayonnaise of Your Very Own

I was surprised to find that making your own mayonnaise is incredibly easy. You'll love the lemony tang that authentic mayonnaise gives to tuna salad, dressings, potato salads, and sandwiches.

Tricks of the Trade

Be careful not to add too much of the oil too quickly; it will separate from the body of the mayonnaise. To fix this, beat in another room-temperature yolk.

Time to the Table: 15 minutes ✤ *Makes 1½ cups*

YOU'LL NEED

2 large egg yolks, beaten until thick

About 1¼ cups vegetable oil

1 tablespoon fresh lemon juice

½ teaspoon dry mustard

½ teaspoon salt

1 tablespoon hot water

1 tablespoon white wine vinegar

Salt and pepper to taste

Let the eggs and oil come to room temperature before starting.

IN A FOOD PROCESSOR OR BLENDER

Combine the lemon juice, mustard, and salt with the eggs. With your food processor pulsing, drizzle in a thin stream of oil, maybe a tablespoon at a time, until the sauce thickens. This will happen after about ½ cup of the oil is added.

Beat in the water and vinegar, and then correct the seasonings with salt, pepper, and lemon juice to taste. Store the mayonnaise in the refrigerator in an impeccably clean container.

Play with Your Food

Mayonnaise is good on its own, but even better as the medium to carry any number of flavors for your foods. Perhaps the most popular in France is aïoli garlic sauce, the "butter of Provence." To make this, soak a piece of dry French bread in a touch of milk until the bread is soggy and then ring it out. Add 2 large egg yolks and, depending on your love of garlic, 3 to 5 garlic cloves, minced, to the bread. Blend, and then add it to the completed mayonnaise recipe above. This is wonderful with boiled potatoes, fish, or with the toast rounds in fish soup.

Try the mayonnaise herbed with chives or scallions, or substitute lime juice for the lemon.

FAUX-FOOD EQUIVALENT: *Hellmann's 97% Fat-Free Mayonnaise*

Ingredients: Water, corn syrup, soybean oil, food starch (modified), egg whites, vinegar, salt, maltodextrin, cellulose gum, xanthan gum, carrageenan, natural flavors, color added, mustard flour, sodium benzoate, calcium disodium EDTA.

Basil Pesto Cream

This is my daughter Grace's favorite sauce. Basil picked from your garden and fresh Parmesan will bring this pesto to life. The pesto is perfect touched over cold summer soup, smeared on a crust of bread, or served with spaghetti.

Time to the Table: 5 minutes ❦ *Makes about 2 cups*

Tricks of the Trade

A food processor works just as well as a mortar and pestle and is quite a bit easier.

YOU'LL NEED

1½ cups packed fresh basil leaves
2 cloves garlic, minced
¾ cup pine nuts
¾ cup grated Parmesan cheese
½ cup extra-virgin olive oil
1 teaspoon heavy cream
Salt and pepper to taste

IN A FOOD PROCESSOR OR BLENDER

Puree all the ingredients until smooth.

Play with Your Food

In summer, try chive pesto. Puree together about a cup of chopped chives with about ¾ cup olive oil, a minced garlic clove, a modest amount of pine nuts, and about ¼ cup of some grated salty cheese.

In winter, when fresh basil is out of season, you can still build a delightful pesto from other ingredients, such as mushrooms or roasted red peppers. All proportions remain as in the recipe above.

FAUX-FOOD EQUIVALENT: *Knorr Creamy Pesto Pasta Sauce*

Ingredients: corn starch, wheat flour, partially hydrogenated soybean oil, salt, maltodextrin, dehydrogenated vegetables, Parmesan cheese, monosodium glutamate, spices, sugar, lactose, disodium phosphate, sodium caseinate.

Sausage Gravy Béchamel

What's the difference between the milk gravy you have over your buttermilk biscuits and a fancy béchamel sauce? Nothing. This gravy is one step better because it's enriched with hot sausage bits and the oil comes from the seasoned drippings of the pork. You really don't need much sausage to add richness.

This goes just fine over toast, but is best over biscuits.

Time to the Table: 15 minutes ✤ Makes about 1 cup

YOU'LL NEED
> About ⅛ cup ground Italian sausage
> 3 tablespoons sausage drippings
> 3 tablespoons all-purpose flour
> 1 cup milk
> Salt and pepper to taste

IN A SKILLET
Fry the sausage over medium heat until done. As it cooks, crumble it up as fine as you can with your spatula.

In a separate pan, add the oil from the sausage (drippings), and then whisk in the flour to make a light roux, making sure the flour is all taken up into the oil. Allow it to slip into a gentle nut-brown color.

Add the milk and stir into a fluid gravy. Stir in the crumbled sausage. Season to taste with salt and pepper, and ladle generously over homemade biscuits.

Play with Your Food

You can use any sausage you want, but sage sausage is excellent.

The color and richness of the gravy depends completely on the roux. Although the standard gravy that never misses is light, you may prefer more complex, darker flavors. If so, let it deepen in color from pale to dark chocolate before adding the milk.

Add a bay leaf, a couple of sage leaves, or a pinch of nutmeg.

FAUX-FOOD EQUIVALENT: *Libby's Country Gravy*

Ingredients: Water, sausage with caramel color, soybean oil, modified food starch, wheat flour, sodium caseinate, salt, sugar, dipotassium phosphate, sodium steroyl lactylate, spice, titanium dioxide, cellulose gum, natural and artificial flavoring.

Garlic-Parmesan Ranch Dressing

My friend Virginia brandished a bottle of ranch salad dressing. "You can't make that yourself, how would you even *start*?" she wondered. The daunting impossibility of the task was resolved, though, when we rummaged through her cabinets and dug out some olive oil, vinegar, mustard, and spices. She had everything she needed already.

It's easy to make something much better than the ready-made store brand.

Time to the Table: 5 minutes ✤ *Makes about 1 cup*

Tricks of the Trade

Raw garlic will lend a strong kick to this dressing. To minimize that effect, make sure it is minced as small as possible.

YOU'LL NEED

 1 cup mayonnaise

 4 tablespoons white wine vinegar

 ¼ cup chopped chives

 1 to 2 cloves garlic, minced

 Freshly ground pepper to taste

 ½ cup grated Parmesan cheese

IN A SMALL BOWL

Mix the mayonnaise and vinegar until smooth, and then add the chives, garlic, and pepper. Sprinkle in the Parmesan, stir to combine, and serve.

Play with Your Food

Cut the vinegar in half and replace it with a squeeze of lemon juice. If the flavor of the mayonnaise is not quite right for you, cut the amount in half and replace it with sour cream.

FAUX-FOOD EQUIVALENT: *Kraft Ranch Dressing Free*

Ingredients: Water, corn syrup, buttermilk, vinegar, onion juice, sugar, garlic juice, salt, modified food starch, soybean oil, xanthan gum, artificial color, phosphoric acid, propylene glycol alginate, monosodium glutamate, potassium sorbate, calcium disodium EDTA, natural flavor, dried parsley, dried green onion, vitamin E acetate, spice, Yellow No. 5, sulfating agents.

"Still Kicking" Barbecue Sauce

Making this barbecue sauce reminds me of the craggy witches in *Macbeth,* hunched over their cauldrons. This recipe doesn't require any toad's ears or rat's claws, but it does call for almost every spice in the cabinet. This happens to be one of the few recipes in this book with more ingredients than the faux food equivalent!

Like any good brew, this sauce definitely qualifies as a Saturday concoction to simmer through the day.

Time to the Table: 1 to 2 hours ❧ *Makes about 6 cups*

YOU'LL NEED

 2 tablespoons extra-virgin olive oil
 1 cup finely minced onion
 3 cloves garlic, minced
 1 hot pepper, such as jalepeño, seeded and minced
 ¼ cup red wine
 2 28-ounce cans tomato sauce
 ½ cup Worcestershire sauce
 ¼ cup cider vinegar
 2 tablespoons molasses
 2 tablespoons Tabasco sauce
 2 tablespoons Dijon mustard
 ¼ cup brown sugar
 1 tablespoon chili powder
 1 teaspoon ground cumin
 5 to 7 turns of a pepper grinder
 Salt to taste

IN A 2-QUART SAUCEPAN

Heat the olive oil over medium heat, add the onion and garlic, and sauté until the onions soften. Throw in the hot pepper and move it around the pan for another couple of minutes. Add the wine, and simmer for 5 minutes before adding the tomato sauce, Worcestershire sauce, cider vinegar, molasses, Tabasco sauce, mustard, brown sugar, chili powder, cumin, pepper, and salt to the pan. Taste at least twice to correct the seasonings.

Bring to a boil, reduce to simmer, and then cover and let it gently stew for an hour or so. It only gets better as it cooks. You can leave it simmering as long as you like, but an hour is about the minimum. Then turn off the heat, cool, and store in a clean leftover ketchup bottle or other container in your refrigerator. It keeps in the refrigerator for 6 to 8 weeks.

Play with Your Food

You can adjust the flavors as you go. It takes a bit of time for a new addition to get infused into the sauce, so what you taste just after the addition won't be exactly how it will taste after another 20 minutes.

FAUX-FOOD EQUIVALENT: *Kraft Original Barbecue Sauce*

Ingredients: High-fructose corn syrup, vinegar, water, concentrated tomato juice, modified food starch, salt, molasses, paprika, spice, mustard flour, caramel color, guar gum, natural flavor, Red No. 40.

Everyday Bacon Bits

In France, you can buy little fatty ham pieces already cut up, called *lardons.* To get the same effect, all you need is a slab of bacon.

You don't need to cook the entire slab at once. Once you slice it into its little pieces, store it in the refrigerator in a Ziploc bag and pull out a few when you are frying something. You can also cook an entire slice of bacon and then crumble it up afterward, if you like it very crispy.

These bacon bits can be used for cream sauces, salads, risottos, omelets, or any dish that needs a little savory flavor.

Tricks of the Trade

When you're cutting your bacon, it's easiest if you cut across the entire slab. If you try to cut up one bacon slice at a time, the slice will tear and you'll never finish.

Time to the Table: 10 minutes   ✤   *Make as much as you need*

YOU'LL NEED

Bacon, thickly sliced

FIRST

Cut your bacon into the number of little ¼-inch pieces you will need for your dish.

IN A MEDIUM SAUCEPAN

Over medium heat, simply cook the bacon until it reaches the desired level of crispness. Remove to a paper towel set on a plate.

FAUX-FOOD EQUIVALENT: *Bac*Os*

Ingredients: Defatted soy flour, partially hydrogenated soybean oil, water, salt, sugar, artificial and natural flavor, Red No. 40 and other color added, soy sauce (water, wheat, soybeans, salt), hydrolyzed vegetable protein (corn, soy, wheat).

Balsamic Vinaigrette Dressing

Time to the Table: 5 minutes ✤ *Makes 1 cup*

YOU'LL NEED

¼ *cup balsamic vinegar*

¾ *cup extra-virgin olive oil*

Spices: some combination of salt, pepper, oregano, garlic powder, cayenne pepper, and parsley to taste

---

Tricks of the Trade

Try adding a touch of Dijon mustard to this dressing. It emulsifies the oil and vinegar into a nice, even consistency.

IN A SMALL MIXING BOWL

Mix the vinegar, olive oil, and spices with a fork. Taste, and correct the seasonings.

Play with Your Food

The classic ratio of oil to vinegar is 3:1. But don't feel bound to this. We like a bit more vinegar in our dressing, especially when it is a good balsamic variety. Also, lemon juice is a good tangy addition to help balance the sweetness of the balsamic. Depending on the kind of veggies you have in your salad, throw some blue cheese into the mix, too.

FAUX-FOOD EQUIVALENT: *Kraft Balsamic Vinaigrette*

Ingredients: Water, canola and/or soybean oil, balsamic vinegar, sugar, salt, dried garlic, spice, xanthan gum, mustard flour, dried parsley, potassium sorbate, calcium disodium EDTA, oleoresin, paprika, sulfating agents.

Double-Almond Biscotti

The word *biscotti* is derived from *bis* (twice) and *cotto* (cooked). Because they are cooked twice, biscotti are dried enough to keep well for quite a long time, without preservatives.

The biscotti you buy in the store are often too dry and crunchy. That's because they were shipped in on a truck from the regional baking facilities in Walla Walla, Washington. But real biscotti resembles a good baguette—a crunch on the outside and a soft, even texture in the middle.

Time to the Table: 90 minutes ✤ *Makes 25 to 30 biscotti*

YOU'LL NEED
½ cup sugar
½ cup (1 stick) unsalted butter, softened
2 large eggs
1¾ cups all-purpose flour
2 teaspoons baking powder
½ teaspoon salt
Pinch of baking soda
¼ teaspoon almond extract
1 cup slivered almonds

Preheat the oven to 350°F.

IN A LARGE MIXING BOWL

Add the sugar and, with an electric blender (or a whisk, a good strong arm, and plenty of patience), cream in the butter and then the eggs. In a separate bowl, mix the flour, baking powder, salt, and baking soda together.

Then fold the dry ingredients into the sugar-butter-egg mixture with a spoon. As you blend these together, add the almond extract and slivered almonds until they're evenly distributed.

Tricks of the Trade

When "oven drying" these biscotti, ten minutes per side in the oven should be enough to keep them moist on the inside. But if your oven tends to cook hot, reduce the heat to 325°F before baking the cut pieces.

ON A LIGHTLY DUSTED BOARD

Knead the dough several minutes and then form it into a broad loaf that will fit your cookie sheet, flattened to about 1½ inches high and 4 inches wide.

Place the dough on an ungreased cookie sheet and bake for 30 minutes. Let cool for 10 minutes on a wire rack. Slice crosswise into ½-inch, biscotti-size pieces.

Place the slices, cut side down, back onto the cookie sheet and bake for 10 minutes. Turn them over and bake on the other side for another 10 minutes. Remove and cool the biscotti on a wire rack.

Play with Your Food

For vanilla biscotti, substitute vanilla extract for the almond extract.

For chocolate-orange biscotti, substitute vanilla extract for the almond extract. Add 1 tablespoon orange juice, 1 teaspoon grated orange rind, and 1 cup bittersweet chocolate shavings or chips. It also wouldn't hurt to throw 2 tablespoons cocoa into the mix.

FAUX-FOOD EQUIVALENT: *The Bake Shop Traditional Almond Biscotti*
Ingredients: Flour, malted barley flour, potassium bromate, sugar, eggs, partially hydrogenated soybean oil and/or cottonseed oil, salt, artificial color and flavor, almonds, baking powder, molasses, natural and/or artificial flavors.

Hot Cocoa

Real hot cocoa is perfect for cold winter evenings when it's late and you don't want a caffeinated drink like coffee or tea, and you don't want to give your kids that packet of hot chocolate mix that has been around since Elvis appeared on *The Ed Sullivan Show.*

Time to the Table: 10 minutes ✤ *Enough for 1 person*

Tricks of the Trade

Be careful heating the cocoa because it scorches easily. Keep your burner at medium or lower.

YOU'LL NEED
1 cup milk
1 heaping tablespoon cocoa powder
1 tablespoon brown sugar
1 teaspoon vanilla extract

IN A MEDIUM SAUCEPAN
Heat the milk over medium heat, and add the cocoa, brown sugar, and vanilla.

Whisk until all the cocoa is incorporated into the milk. Heat the milk until just steamy, stirring all the while.

Play with Your Food
If you don't have cocoa, simply substitute 1 to 2 squares of chopped bittersweet chocolate. Warm the chocolate slowly and whisk in ¼ cup

of the milk until thoroughly melted. Then continue with the rest of the recipe.

For fancy hot cocoa, add a pinch of cinnamon and top with a healthy dollop of whipped cream, sprinkled with finely shaved chocolate.

FAUX-FOOD EQUIVALENT: *Nestlé Rich Chocolate Hot Cocoa Mix*

Ingredients: Sugar, corn syrup solids, dairy product solids, vegetable oil (partially hydrogenated coconut and palm kernel oils, canola, hydrogenated palm, soybean, cottonseed or safflower oils), cocoa processed with alkali, cellulose gum, salt, sodium caseinate, dipotassium phosphate, sodium silicoaluminate, mono- and diglycerides, guar gum, artificial flavors.

Buttered Popcorn

On movie night number one, start with the microwave popcorn you picked up to go with your movie. Open up the plastic packaging and take the bag over to the microwave. Put it in and set the timer for 4 minutes. On movie night number two, take a jar of popcorn and pour some into an oiled pan. Turn on the heat and wait 4 minutes, while you melt some butter in the microwave.

The only real difference between these two approaches is a pan to wash. The second method replaces heart-clogging hydrogenated oils with real butter—which contains vitamins and minerals.

Time to the Table: 10 minutes ✦ *Makes 2 to 3 cups*

Tricks of the Trade

To prevent burning the popcorn: Once the corn starts popping, hold either side of the pan with pot holders and shuffle it back and forth to the rhythm of whatever song you are listening to. This serves a dual purpose. It also ensures that all the kernels sift to the bottom to be popped.

YOU'LL NEED

Enough vegetable oil to cover the bottom of a saucepan
½ cup popcorn kernels
2 tablespoons unsalted butter
Salt to taste

IN A MEDIUM SAUCEPAN

Add the oil until it just barely covers the entire bottom of the pan, then pour in the popcorn until it forms a single layer. Cover.

Heat the popcorn over medium-high heat until the first kernels start to pop. Then shake the pan until the number of pops is fewer than 1 every 2 seconds. Pour the popcorn into a large serving or mixing bowl.

Melt the butter in a separate pan or in the microwave. Pour the melted butter over the top of the popcorn in a thin stream, making sure the corn is evenly coated by tossing it around at the same time.

Play with Your Food

Infuse your butter with garlic or rosemary by warming 1 crushed garlic clove or ⅛ teaspoon dried rosemary in the melted butter for about 2 minutes. You might also try adding just a few crushed walnuts or almonds to the popcorn as well.

Other suggestions for popcorn include grating some hard cheese such as Parmesan very fine and sprinkling it all over after the butter is tossed in.

FAUX-FOOD EQUIVALENT: *Pop-Secret Popcorn*

Ingredients: Popcorn, partially hydrogenated soybean oil, salt, butter, artificial and natural flavors, color added, propyl gallate.

Brown Sugar Cinnamon Oatmeal

This oatmeal tastes so good that it's hard to believe how good it is for you. The insoluble fiber found in this hearty breakfast can help reduce the risk of heart disease and lower your LDL cholesterol.

Time to the Table: 10 minutes ✤ *Serves 1*

YOU'LL NEED

1 cup water

½ cup rolled oats

Pinch of salt

1 tablespoon unsalted butter

1 tablespoon brown sugar

½ teaspoon ground cinnamon

IN A MEDIUM SAUCEPAN

Boil the water, then add the oats and salt. Lower the heat to medium and cook until the water is absorbed (for whole oats, about 15 minutes; for quick oats, 5 to 10 minutes). Add the butter, brown sugar, and cinnamon. Correct the seasonings.

Play with Your Food

Add any fruit: whole, sliced thinly, or quickly pureed with a touch of sugar.

Replace the brown sugar with maple syrup and add a touch of pure cream.

FAUX-FOOD EQUIVALENT: *Quaker Instant Strawberries and Cream Oatmeal*

Ingredients: Oats, sugar, maltodextrin, partially hydrogenated soybean oil, whey, sodium caseinate, dehydrated apples treated with sodium sulfite, artificial strawberry flavor, citric acid, Red No. 40, salt, calcium carbonate, guar gum, artificial flavors, citric acid, niacinamide, vitamin A palmitate, reduced iron, pyridoxine hydrochloride, riboflavin, thiamin, mononitrate, folic acid.

Banana Nut Pancakes

A staple of Saturday mornings, these pancakes are easy to throw together and very versatile.

Time to the Table: 15 minutes ❧ *Makes 9 to 12 pancakes*

Tricks of the Trade

You can make only a few pancakes at a time. So, to allow your family to eat all together, put a large plate in a warm oven (150°F) and set the pancakes on it until they're all made and you're ready for everyone to eat.

YOU'LL NEED

1 large egg, beaten

¾ to 1 cup milk (see below)

1 cup all-purpose flour

2 tablespoons vegetable oil, plus more for the griddle

3 teaspoons baking powder

1 tablespoon brown sugar

Pinch of salt

Pinch of ground cinnamon

1 pungent ripe banana, mashed until smooth

1 cup crushed walnuts

IN A LARGE MIXING BOWL

Beat the egg and milk (if you like your pancakes thick, use less milk; play with the amount to make your perfect pancakes) together, then add the flour and mix until smooth. Fold in the oil, baking powder, brown sugar, salt, cinnamon, banana, and walnuts.

TO A FRYING PAN OR GRIDDLE

Add about a tablespoon of oil and place it over medium heat. Then add about ¼ cup of the batter to the pan. You can vary this amount depending on the size of the pancakes you prefer. Look to see when the batter develops bubbles, indicating the underside is golden. When ready, give it a flip and repeat the process for the other side.

Play with Your Food

Try sliced strawberries or blueberries instead of bananas.

These pancakes are just as good with maple syrup and butter as they are with some all-fruit jelly and whipped cream.

FAUX-FOOD EQUIVALENT: *Mrs. Butterworth's Complete Pancake and Waffle Mix*

Ingredients: Wheat flour, sugar, leavening (baking soda, sodium aluminum phosphate, monocalcium phosphate), soy flour, whey, dextrose, partially hydrogenated soybean and cottonseed oils, salt, whole eggs, calcium carbonate, soy protein isolate, nonfat milk, sodium caseinate, mono- and diglycerides, natural and artificial flavors (includes dairy derivatives), caramel color.

Quick Ham and Egg Scramble

You will never in your wildest dreams imagine the behemoth of a faux-food-ingredients list for what should be a simple ham and egg scramble or omelet. Check out the faux food below, but I warn you: It's ugly.

Instead, a few real foods make for a fabulously easy Saturday breakfast that takes a few minutes to cook.

Time to the Table: 10 to 15 minutes ❦ *Serves 2*

YOU'LL NEED
> 2 tablespoons unsalted butter
> ¼ cup fully cooked diced ham
> ¼ cup diced sweet red bell pepper
> Salt and freshly ground pepper to taste
> 4 large eggs, beaten

IN A LARGE FRYING PAN

Melt the butter over medium heat, add the ham and red pepper, and sauté until just barely done (about 2 minutes), as they'll cook a bit more along with the eggs. Season with salt and pepper to taste. Add the beaten eggs, keeping the heat on medium, and thoroughly mix the ham and pepper through the eggs. Cook until the eggs are as firm as you like them.

Play with Your Food

Clean out your fridge. Everything works in this—onions, spinach, bacon (of course), potatoes, mushrooms, tomatoes (sun-dried tomatoes are fantastic), or smoked salmon. Sprinkle in some Parmesan or goat cheese to hold it all together.

You could also add 1 teaspoon of cream to your beaten eggs—it's wonderful.

FAUX-FOOD EQUIVALENT: *Uncle Ben's Breakfast Bowl, Ham, Eggs, and Peppers*

Ingredients: Scrambled eggs (whole eggs, skim milk, soybean oil, modified food starch, salt, xanthan gum, liquid pepper extract, citric acid, natural and artificial butter flavor [clarified butter, lipolyzed butter oil, artificial flavor, annatto]), potatoes (sodium acid pyrophosphate, water), fully cooked diced ham (cured with water, salt, sugar, sodium phosphates, sodium erythorbate, sodium nitrate), green bell peppers, red bell peppers, onions, reduced-fat cheddar cheese (pasteurized part-skim milk, cheese culture, salt, enzymes, annatto, vitamin A palmitate [calcium carbonate, potato starch, powdered cellulose]), nonfat dry milk, lightly salted butter, chicken base (roast chicken, chicken fat, autolyzed yeast extract, gelatin, maltodextrin, salt, chicken broth, flavoring [contains torula yeast], sugar, dehydrated mushrooms, xanthan gum), modified corn starch, bacon base (cooked bacon [cured with water, salt, sodium phosphate, sugar, sodium erythorbate, and nitrate]), salt, yeast extract, ham stock, bacon fat (TBHQ, citric acid), sugar, corn starch, natural flavorings, natural smoke flavorings, caramel coloring, potassium sorbate, corn syrup solids, natural butter flavor (whey, natural flavors, salt, corn syrup solids, guar gum, annatto, turmeric extract), stabilizer (modified food starch, xanthan gum, guar gum), onion powder, black pepper.

Tilapia with Sherry and Rosemary

Tricks of the Trade

To make sure the fish is cooked all the way through, notice when the center responds to gentle prodding by flaking apart. That's when you're ready to pull it out and eat!

Time to the Table: 15 minutes ✤ *Serves 3*

YOU'LL NEED

> *3 small tilapia fillets*
> *Salt and freshly ground pepper to taste*
> *¼ cup extra-virgin olive oil*
> *4 cloves garlic, minced*
> *2 tablespoons fresh rosemary*
> *Pinch of cayenne pepper*
> *¾ cup dry sherry*

Season the fish with salt and pepper and set aside.

IN A MEDIUM PAN

Heat the olive oil over medium heat, then sauté the garlic and 1½ tablespoons of the rosemary for a couple of minutes, until the garlic just starts to brown.

ADD THE FILLETS

Setting them side by side in the pan, sprinkle with some of the cayenne and remaining rosemary. After 3 minutes, flip the fillets and sprinkle with the cayenne and rosemary again. Continue to cook until done through (about 4 minutes).

PREPARE THE SAUCE

Remove the fish to a warm plate and add the sherry to the pan, deglazing by scraping up the bits of fish and garlic from the bottom of the pan. Cook these drippings over medium-high heat until reduced by more than half and the sauce is almost syrupy (about 4 to 5 minutes). Serve the sauce hot over the fillets.

Play with Your Food

Thyme is another great seasoning to go with fish and can be substituted for the rosemary. Add a tang to the mix by sautéing a little lime zest with the garlic at the beginning or by squeezing lime juice over the fish.

FAUX-FOOD EQUIVALENT: *Swanson Breaded Fish Fillet*

Ingredients: Alaska pollock, bleached wheat flour, partially hydrogenated soybean oil, water, modified food starch, salt, dextrose, corn flour, yeast, malt syrup, sugar, cellulose gum, soy flour, carrageenan, oleoresin, paprika, spice, leavening (sodium acid pyrophosphate, sodium bicarbonate), mono- and diglycerides, natural flavor, sodium alginate.

The Last Lasagna

Lasagna underachievers come in many varieties. The worst of the bunch are those with oversugared sauce. The second is the flavorless kind that some restaurants serve because they've got to lower the bar for the masses. Some patrons don't like it seasoned, so no one gets it seasoned.

If you have a favorite place to get your lasagna, please don't make this one. It's so good, it's the last lasagna you'll ever try.

Time to the Table: 1 hour ✤ *Serves 15 to 18*

Tricks of the Trade

When cooking the noodles, be sure to put the olive oil in the water. Otherwise, after you strain them, they'll dry out, stick together, and tear.

If you have problems with acidic foods, place a couple of carrot slices in the sauce while it cooks.

FOR THE SAUCE YOU'LL NEED

1 pound spicy Italian sausage

1 medium onion, chopped

4 garlic cloves, minced

1 28-ounce can diced tomatoes

1 15-ounce can tomato sauce

Salt and freshly ground pepper to taste

1 or 2 bay leaves

1 teaspoon dried oregano

1 teaspoon dried basil

Pinch of cayenne pepper

½ cup red wine

FOR THE RICOTTA CHEESE MIX YOU'LL NEED

1 16-ounce container ricotta cheese

1 large egg

¼ cup grated Parmesan cheese

Salt and freshly ground pepper to taste

1 teaspoon dried oregano

12 lasagna noodles

1 pound whole-milk mozzarella cheese, grated

Cook 12 lasagna noodles in a pan of salted boiling water and a splash of olive oil.

MAKE THE SAUCE

In a large pan over medium heat, cook the Italian sausage with the onion and garlic until browned. Add the tomatoes and tomato sauce right to the pan. Add the salt, pepper, bay leaves, oregano, basil, cayenne, and red wine. Simmer for at least 10 minutes. Taste and adjust the seasonings.

The sauce can simmer over low heat for a while, because it only gets better as it cooks. While the sauce is bubbling its way into its various stages of perfection, continue with the lasagna.

MAKE THE RICOTTA CHEESE MIX

In a large bowl, mix the ricotta, egg, Parmesan, salt, pepper, and oregano. Use your own discretion here. You may be reading this recipe and thinking, "A quarter cup Parmesan? Only ¼ cup Parmesan?" If so, throw in some more.

Preheat the oven to 350° F.

IN A STANDARD LASAGNA PAN

Line the bottom of the pan with lasagna noodles. Spread a third of the ricotta mix onto the pasta, and a third of the sauce over the ricotta mix. Sprinkle a third of the mozzarella onto the sauce. Repeat the process for the remaining 2 layers ingredients.

IN THE OVEN

Bake for 45 minutes. When the cheese is crisping a bit on the top and the sauce is bubbling up on the sides, pull it out. If you can resist it, allow another 30 minutes for it to cool and set.

FAUX-FOOD EQUIVALENT: *Marie Callender's Meat Lasagna*

Ingredients: Tomatoes (water, tomato paste), lasagna pasta (water, enriched semolina), ricotta cheese (pasteurized whey, milk, cream), seasoned cooked beef (beef, seasoning [flavorings, salt, spices, dextrose], tomato paste, salt, soybean oil), premium pizza cheese (part-skim mozzarella [pasteurized part-skim milk, cheese cultures, whey protein concentrate, enzymes]), Parmesan and Romano cheese (part-skim milk, cheese culture, salt, enzymes, cellulose powder [to prevent caking]), garlic (contains citric acid), carrots, celery, seasoning (salt, dextrose, sugar, spice, spice extractives, disodium inosinate, and disodium guanylate [flavor enhancer], tricalcium phosphate and soybean oil), onions, heavy whipping cream, sugar, salt, bread crumbs (wheat flour, sugar, partially hydrogenated soybean oil, salt, yeast, and calcium propionate), spices, modified food starch, dried egg whites.

Red Roasted Chicken

Roasted chicken makes for dozens of delicious dishes. After you have the bird itself for dinner, you can pull the leftover meat off the bones for a stir-fry, Chicken Potpie in Sherry Cream Sauce (page 283), stews, salads, and barbecues. Save the chicken bones to make Super Chicken Stock (page 290). This stock makes any soup better, any sauce richer, and any risotto irresistible.

Because the chicken is covered while baked, the overall flavor is infused by the red wine and herbs you add beforehand.

Tricks of the Trade

Keeping the chicken covered is a great way to keep it from drying out because, essentially, it bastes itself.

Time to the Table: 50 minutes ⚜ *Serves 6*

YOU'LL NEED

1 medium whole chicken, washed and patted dry

1 tablespoon extra-virgin olive oil

Salt and freshly ground pepper to taste

¼ cup red wine vinegar

¼ cup red wine

1 medium onion, coarsely chopped

5 to 10 whole, peeled garlic cloves

BEFORE YOU BAKE

Preheat the oven to 400° F. Place the chicken in a baking pan lined with aluminum foil. Rub it with the olive oil and give it a good sprinkle of salt and pepper. Simply add the vinegar, red wine, onion, and garlic to the pan. Enclose the chicken with aluminum foil, and place in the oven for 40 minutes.

AFTER IT'S DONE

Pull out the chicken and remove the upper layer of foil from the pan. Turn the temperature to broil, put the pan back in the oven, and brown the chicken skin for about 5 minutes.

Play with Your Food

The juices in the bottom of the pan can be seasoned as you like, with lime juice or with 2 tablespoons each of honey and spicy mustard. Or you can make it Mediterranean by adding capers and olives to the base of the pan.

And please experiment with the vegetables. Carrots and potatoes will add a little sweetness to the broth.

FAUX-FOOD EQUIVALENT: *Healthy Choice Country Herb Chicken*

Ingredients: Chicken breast with rib meat, water, soy protein isolate, modified food starch, chicken seasoning (modified food starch, dextrose, paprika, spice, xanthan gum), salt, chicken flavor (autolyzed yeast extract, chicken flavor [maltodextrin, natural flavor, mono- and diglycerides], salt, chicken fat, citric acid), partially hydrogenated soybean oil, sodium tri-polyphosphate, flavoring, gravy (water, sherry [sulfating agents], modified food starch, cream, flavorings [including clam extract], soybean oil, rice starch, nonfat milk, salt, chicken powder, spices, autolyzed yeast extract, sodium caseinate, caramel color, maltodextrin, chicken fat, partially hydrogenated soybean and/or cottonseed oil, turmeric, beef extract, citric acid, mushroom powder), roasted potatoes (potatoes, soybean oil, salt, maltodextrin, wheat starch, dehydrated onion, sugar, red bell pepper, corn starch, parsley, paprika, spices, flavor, caramel color, garlic, turmeric extract, annatto extract, citric acid), water, cherries, broccoli, cauliflower, carrots, brown sugar, cherry juice, rolled oats, modified starch, sugar, cream, crisped rice (rice flour, sugar, malt, salt, glycerol monosterate, rice extract), soybean oil, partially hydrogenated soybean oil, honey, brown sugar, molasses, corn syrup, spices, sodium steroyl lactilate (emulsifier), salt, almond oil, alcohol, butter oil, enzyme-modified butter fat, dried whey, nonfat dry milk, soy lecithin (emulsifier), corn oil, vitamin A palmitate, beta carotene.

Chicken Potpie in Sherry Cream Sauce

Time to the Table: 60 minutes ❦ *Serves 8*

Tricks of the Trade

You don't want the vegetables in your potpie to turn to mush, even though you're going to cook them twice. So make sure to undercook your vegetables at first, because they'll be baked in the pie itself for 45 minutes.

YOU'LL NEED

> *1 piecrust with top and bottom*
> *2 tablespoons plus ¼ cup (½ stick) unsalted butter*
> *½ cup chopped onion*
> *½ cup chopped carrots*
> *½ cup chopped celery*
> *½ cup sliced mushrooms*
> *2 cups chopped cooked chicken*
> *½ cup all-purpose flour*
> *2 cups chicken stock*
> *3 tablespoons dry sherry*
> *1 tablespoon minced fresh rosemary or 1 teaspoon dried*
> *1 cup half-and-half*
> *Salt and freshly ground pepper to taste*

Preheat the oven to 425° F.

IN A LARGE SAUCEPAN

In 1 tablespoon of butter, sauté the onion, carrots, celery, and mushrooms over medium heat until they just soften, then remove from the pan. Sauté the chicken in a second tablespoon of butter until browned, but not crisp, and remove from the pan.

Over medium heat, add the remaining butter, and then the flour. Stir until the roux is chestnut brown. Add the chicken stock and whisk until all the roux is incorporated.

Bring this mixture to a boil, reduce to a simmer, and add the sherry, rosemary, half-and-half, and salt and pepper. Taste and correct the seasonings. After the broth has become quite thick, fold in the vegetables and chicken and continue to heat for 10 minutes.

IN THE OVEN

Pour the potpie filling into the pie plate with the crust on the bottom, and top with the second layer of crust. Be sure to press the two crusts together along the edges to form a good seal. Bake for 30 minutes, until crust is golden. Serve right away, but be careful, it's hot.

Play with Your Food

The vegetables you choose are absolutely up to you. Potatoes also go perfectly in this dish. Just dice and sauté along with the other vegetables early on in the recipe.

You will taste the rosemary right away, but another savory alternative is sage.

If you don't have sherry, try a port wine instead. Once you have the basics of this recipe, you can modify it any way you choose!

FAUX-FOOD EQUIVALENT: *Pepperidge Farm Pot Pie with Chicken*

Ingredients: Chicken stock, unbleached enriched wheat flour, roasted white chicken meat, water, partially hydrogenated vegetable shortening (soybean and cottonseed oils, colored with beta-carotene), carrots, peas, green beans, corn cream, modified food starch, chicken fat, caseinates (whey, calcium, and sodium), enriched bleached wheat flour, salt, pie dough base (dextrose, gelatinized wheat starch, salt, baking soda, calcium propionate [preservative], partially hydrogenated soybean and/or cottonseed oil, sodium bisulfite), dextrose, natural flavoring, garlic juice, onion juice, chicken flavor (ascorbic acid, salt, chicken stock, chicken powder, chicken fat), sodium phosphate, soy protein isolate, sugar, caramel color, disodium guanylate, disodium inosinate, corn syrup, citric acid, spice extract, spice, oleoresin, turmeric, corn oil, beta-carotene.

Crock-Pot Beef Stew

Crock-Pots make for the easiest kind of cooking: You can handle dinner and do something else at the same time. Even better, the long, slow cooking process makes the meat so tender it falls apart.

Tricks of the Trade

Judge how long you want the cooking to last. If you are just getting started at two in the afternoon, put the Crock-Pot temperature on high. If you're going to be out for the entire day, put it on low.

Time to the Table: 5 to 7 hours ✤ Serves 14 to 16

YOU'LL NEED

2 tablespoons extra-virgin olive oil

2 pounds rump roast

2 cups hearty red wine

½ teaspoon salt

⅛ teaspoon freshly ground pepper

1 cup chopped onion

1 cup chopped carrots

2 cloves garlic, minced

2 cups beef stock (no MSG)

1 bay leaf

1 teaspoon dried thyme

1 teaspoon cayenne pepper

IN A HEAVY SAUCEPAN

Over medium-high heat, add the olive oil and braise the beef until browned on all sides. Remove the beef to the Crock-Pot, and pour in ½ cup of the red wine to deglaze the pan. Once all the beef bits have been lifted from the pan, pour the contents into the Crock-Pot.

INTO THE CROCK-POT

Add the salt, pepper, onion, carrots, garlic, stock, remaining wine, bay leaf, thyme, and cayenne. Cover and set the temperature to low, go to work, and dream of the heavenly dinner you will have that evening.

When you get home, lift the lid and allow the liquid to cook down a bit while you're getting the rest of dinner ready. Before serving, sample the juices and season with salt and pepper to taste.

Play with Your Food

A few bits of bacon make a wonderful addition to this stew. You don't need more than five or six one-inch pieces, but they really enrich the broth.

If you like a thicker gravy, simply pour the juices into a saucepan and whisk in a mixture of 2 tablespoons softened butter and 2 tablespoons flour for every 2 cups of liquid. This is better than cornstarch, because it thickens and enriches the broth at the same time.

FAUX-FOOD EQUIVALENT: *Banquet Crock-Pot Classics Beef Stew*

Ingredients: Potatoes (potatoes, sodium acid pyrophosphate), cooked diced beef (beef, salt, rosemary extract), carrots, water, onions, seasoning (modified corn starch, hydrolyzed vegetable protein [corn, soy, wheat, autolyzed wheat extract, dextrose]), dehydrated potato, dehydrated onion and garlic, sugar, wheat flour, monosodium glutamate, caramel color, spice (contains sulfites), celery, beef fat (beef fat with BHT and citric acid), beef flavor (beef extract, flavors, autolyzed yeast, salt), salt, potassium chloride, soy lethicin, mono- and diglycerides with DATEM (diacetyl tartaric esters of monoglycerides).

Braised Orange Chicken

This recipe was discovered by accident, after we realized that we were completely out of the usual ingredients—apples and avocados. But this adaptation worked very well.

Time to the Table: 60 minutes ✤ Serves 4

Tricks of the Trade

If there's too much oil in the pan from the chicken, olive oil, etc., the gravy will separate, so be sure to add the water.

A wonderful way to thicken your gravy is to mix equal parts of flour and butter Into a paste (say 1 tablespoon of each) and whisk it into the mix. If the mixture becomes too thick, just add more half-and-half.

YOU'LL NEED

1 tablespoon extra-virgin olive oil

1 tablespoon unsalted butter

1 medium chicken, cut into 4 pieces

1 navel orange, peeled and cut into modest chunks

2 to 3 tablespoons triple sec liqueur

1 to 2 tablespoons water

2 large sprigs rosemary

1 cup half-and-half

Salt and freshly ground pepper to taste

IN A LARGE LIDDED POT

Over medium-high heat, add the olive oil and butter. When the butter is just melted, place the chicken in the pot to braise for about 5 minutes. Turn the pieces to brown the other side for five minutes or so.

Add the orange chunks and triple sec. Very carefully, immediately light a match to it and allow it to burn down. Add the water and 1 sprig of the rosemary, reduce the heat to medium-low, and cover.

Allow this to percolate for about 45 minutes, turning the chicken perhaps once in the middle of the process.

FOR THE GRAVY

Remove the chicken pieces to a warm platter. Proceed with the gravy by increasing the heat to medium-high, and boiling the cooking liquid until it reduces by half, about 3 minutes. During this process, be sure to scrape up the chicken bits on the bottom of the pan with a wooden spoon.

Add the half-and-half and the remaining rosemary sprig. Allow to bubble away for another two to three minutes, and then season with salt and pepper to taste. Serve warm over the chicken, but especially over mashed potatoes.

Play with Your Food

Apple and mushroom is another combination that works very well. Instead of oranges, add a chopped tart apple and flame it with calvados. While the pot is covered, sauté sliced mushrooms (darker varieties are tastier) and add into the sauce at the end.

FAUX-FOOD EQUIVALENT: *McCormick's Chicken Gravy Mix*

Ingredients: Wheat flour, modified wheat starch, dextrose, salt, whey solids, monosodium glutamate, chicken meat, chicken fat, silicon dioxide, onion, chicken broth, xanthan gum, chicken skin, yeast extract, spice, natural flavor, paprika, disodium inosinate, disodium guanylate, FD&C Yellow No. 5, FD&C Yellow No. 6, soy sauce.

Tricks of the Trade

Cook this dish with the lid off the pot. This will concentrate the flavor in the juices, which you'll notice right away when you serve a little extra to douse your rice with.

Pork and Beans

This delicious comfort food can't be beat for warm, homey flavor. The beans emerge with the nutty taste and texture of boiled peanuts. If you've never been to the South and nibbled on boiled peanuts, here's your chance to try the flavor without having to make the trip.

Time to the Table: 3 to 4 hours ✤ *Serves 15 to 18*

YOU'LL NEED

    1 16-ounce bag pinto beans, rinsed

    2 quarts water

    1 cup chopped onion

    ½ pound pork ribs

    3 cloves garlic, minced

    3 bay leaves

    3 rosemary sprigs or 1 tablespoon dried rosemary

    2 tablespoons salt

    1 tablespoon pepper

TO A CROCK-POT

Add all the ingredients, turn the Crock-Pot on high, and leave all day long, until the beans are barely done. If cooking on the stove, add all the ingredients to a large stockpot, bring to a boil, and then simmer with the lid on until the beans are just soft (about 90 minutes).

Play with Your Food

This dish is wonderful with rice, some Tabasco sauce, and hot sausage on the side. Add a beer and you have perfect game-day food. If you don't want to use pork ribs, spicy sausage will work just as well.

Add a pinch of allspice or cumin to give it more of a Jamaican twist. I also love the Cajun flavor that gumbo filé gives to beans.

FAUX-FOOD EQUIVALENT: *Campbell's Pork and Beans*

Ingredients: Water, pea beans, high-fructose corn syrup, modified food starch, salt, tomato puree, distilled vinegar, oleoresin paprika, caramel color, flavoring.

Super Chicken Stock

Although the little cubes of chicken-flavored MSG ought to come with an FDA warning label, for a long time the thought of making my own chicken stock and storing it in the freezer seemed so time consuming. How much better could mine be to justify the time and energy? Given that I am putting this chicken stock recipe in this book, you probably already know the answer. The difference this stock made in my French Onion Soup (page 292), for instance, was stunning.

Make everything possible from this intense stock because its flavor drastically improves everything from sauces and risottos to chicken potpie—once you try it, you can't go back to the cubes. Soon chicken stock becomes the reason to have baked chicken, instead of the other way around.

Time to the Table: At least 3 hours ✤ *Makes 2 quarts*

Tricks of the Trade

Don't boil the stock over very high heat. This makes it cloudy. A simple simmer with the lid off is all you need.

The main trick to this stock is time. It takes a while to concentrate the savory flavors of the chicken and vegetables. That's why we start with 3 quarts of water so we can end up with 2 quarts of stock.

YOU'LL NEED

Carcass of 1 baked chicken

3 quarts water

4 stalks celery, chopped

1 cup chopped carrots

2 cups chopped onion

2 tablespoons salt

3 bay leaves

4 cloves garlic, smashed

5 sage leaves or 2 teaspoons rubbed sage

Several turns of a pepper grinder, to taste

PREPARE THE CHICKEN

After you've had a baked chicken one evening, pick the majority of the meat off and cut the bones into 2-inch pieces.

IN A 4-QUART STOCKPOT

Add the chicken bones with the water and bring to a boil. Once the foam comes to the top, skim it away and add the celery, carrots, onion, salt, bay leaves, garlic, sage, and pepper.

Let it bubble away uncovered for half a day or so, until it cooks down by about a third.

STORING

Strain the stock, let it cool, and store it in a Tupperware container in the refrigerator if you are going to use it within a week. Otherwise, store it in the freezer, where it will keep for up to 3 months.

Play with Your Food

Any number of vegetables go quite nicely into the stock base, although what French Cajuns call the "holy trinity" of vegetables—onion, carrot, and celery—are required staples in any variation.

The best, though, is the addition of a few ginger coins to the broth, which gives it a light lemony flavor.

FAUX-FOOD EQUIVALENT: *Gia Russa Clear Chicken Broth*

Ingredients: Chicken broth, chicken fat, salt, dextrose, seasoning (hydrolyzed soy, corn gluten, wheat gluten proteins, onion powder, modified corn starch, torula yeast, autolyzed yeast, natural flavor, garlic powder, disodium inosinate, disodium guanylate, soybean oil, thiamine hydrochloride, tartaric acid, gum arabic), monosodium glutamate, oleoresin carrot.

French Onion Soup

French onion soup is a dish that proves there's an elegant genius to creating something out of even the most mundane ingredients. From the lowly onion, butter, flour, and cheese, this rich, delicious hot meal in a bowl emerges.

Tricks of the Trade

As in other matters of the skillet, time and flavor trade off. Leave the onions over medium heat and let them slowly sauté, to mellow the floury taste.

Likewise, after the stock goes in, allow the soup its full 40-minute covered cooking time. You'll appreciate the results in the end.

Time to the Table: 1 hour ✤ *Serves 6 to 8*

YOU'LL NEED

1 medium sweet onion, thinly sliced

3 tablespoons unsalted butter

2 tablespoons all-purpose flour

2 quarts chicken stock

2 tablespoons Emmentaler or Swiss cheese per person

1 baguette toast round per person

IN A SKILLET

Sauté the onion in the butter over a gentle medium heat until it softens (a good 15 minutes). Sprinkle in the flour and stir for another 2 minutes.

Add in the chicken stock. Bring to a boil, and then simmer, with the lid on, for 40 minutes.

READY THE REMAINING PARTS

As the soup cooks, grate the cheese, and then toast the bread (baguettes, not surprisingly, work best for this). Simply ladle the broth into oven-safe bowls, top with the toast, and sprinkle with enough cheese to just cover the bread. Broil until the cheese wants to be golden and the soup bubbles up the side of the dish.

Play with Your Food

For a heartier soup, add some sliced mushrooms and chicken meat just after the flour is added. The smokiness of the mushrooms and the heartiness of the chicken are truly delicious and make this soup its own meal.

FAUX-FOOD EQUIVALENT: *Campbell's French Onion Soup*

Ingredients: Onions, beef stock, salt, yeast extract, vegetable oil, potato starch, water, monosodium glutamate, caramel color, hydrolyzed yeast protein, enzyme modified cheddar cheese, beef fat, hydrolyzed soy protein, citric acid, spice extract, dextrose, hydrolyzed wheat gluten.

Tarragon Tuna Salad

This salad is an absolutely delicious rendition of an old standby. Whether you're on the beach, at a picnic, or in your home, this dish stands out on a Saturday afternoon.

Time to the Table: 5 minutes ✤ *Serves 2*

YOU'LL NEED

　　1 can tuna packed in water
　　1 tablespoon mayonnaise
　　1 teaspoon spicy mustard

continued

Capers, to taste
½ teaspoon fresh tarragon
Salt, pepper, and cayenne pepper to taste

Drain the water from the tuna.

IN A MEDIUM MIXING BOWL

Mix the tuna with the mayonnaise, mustard, capers, tarragon, salt, pepper, and cayenne. Taste and fix the flavors to your liking.

Play with Your Food

After you do this once, don't follow the precise ratio of ingredients anymore. This isn't a chemistry experiment; it's an exercise in flavor preference. Don't fit your tastes to the recipe; fit the recipe to your tastes! For an open-faced tuna melt, lightly butter both sides of a bread slice, and brown each side over medium heat. As the second side browns, place sliced Cheddar cheese on the toast to melt. When the cheese softens, add a slice of tomato, a smear of mayonnaise, salt/pepper/oregano to taste, and then tuna over the top. Try this with goat cheese and you'll be hooked for good.

FAUX-FOOD EQUIVALENT: *Chicken of the Sea Mayonnaise and Onion Tuna Salad Kit*

Ingredients: Soybean oil, water, eggs, white vinegar, dehydrated onion, high-fructose corn syrup, salt, spice, xanthan gum, potassium sorbate and sodium benzoate, calcium disodium EDTA, tuna (light tuna, water, vegetable broth, salt), bread crumbs (wheat flour, dextrose, salt, yeast), dried vegetables (diced bell peppers, dried celery, dried onion, sodium bisulfite).

Healthful Pepperoni Pizza

Pizza *can* be a health food when made with natural ingredients: bread, tomatoes, cheese, fresh vegetables, and spices. This recipe is delicious and couldn't be simpler.

Time to the Table: 90 minutes ❦ *Serves 6*

YOU'LL NEED

3 tablespoons olive oil, divided

3 cloves garlic, minced

1 16-ounce can tomato sauce

Sturdy pinches to your liking of basil, oregano, salt, and pepper

¼ cup hearty red wine

1 teaspoon instant yeast

1 teaspoon sugar

1 cup warm water

2½ cups all-purpose flour

1 cup grated mozzarella cheese

25 pepperoni slices

FOR THE SAUCE

In a medium saucepan, heat 1 tablespoon of the olive oil and sauté the garlic for just a few minutes before adding in the tomato sauce, spices, and wine. Let this barely simmer for 10 minutes before correcting the seasonings. Let it simmer for another 15 minutes.

Tricks of the Trade

When the pizza comes bubbling out of the oven, it is very helpful to place it on a large wire rack—much like cookies—so that the bottom becomes crisp.

FOR THE CRUST

In a large mixing bowl, dissolve the yeast and sugar into the warm water for 5 minutes. Mix in the flour, add the remaining 2 tablespoons of olive oil, and mix until smooth. Check to see if it is too dry or too wet. A perfect dough should be just barely sticky. If too dry, add another tablespoon of water. Knead for a minute or two on a lightly dusted board and then set into a clean, oiled mixing bowl. Set in a warm place to rise for 1 hour.

ASSEMBLE THE PIZZA

Preheat the oven to 450° F.

Deflate the dough and roll it out onto a floured board with a rolling pin to make it the shape you like. Be sure to build up the edges so your sauce and goodies don't leak off the sides. Place the dough on a pizza stone or pan and set in the oven for 5 minutes. Remove from the oven and spread on the sauce, cheese, pepperoni, and any other toppings you have.

Reduce the oven temperature to 425° F. Return the pizza to the oven and bake for about 20 minutes. Pull it out when the cheese is golden.

Play with Your Food

Thinly sliced onions are great on pizza, as are all the usual suspects, such as sausage, peppers, and mushrooms.

Another smart adaptation: instead of making one big giant pizza, make several smaller "personal" pizzas that you can use for lunches. This allows everyone to doctor their pizzas to their own tastes.

FAUX-FOOD EQUIVALENT: *Red Baron Pepperoni Pizza*

Ingredients: Crust (flour, water, sugar, soybean oil, corn meal, yeast, partially hydrogenated oil with soy lecithin, TBHQ, citric acid, glucono-delta-lactone, encapsulated sodium bicarbonate, wheat gluten, salt, DATEM), toppings (low-moisture part-skim mozzarella cheese, tomato paste, water, pepperoni [pork, beef, salt, water, paprika, dextrose, natural spices, smoke flavoring, lactic acid starter culture, sodium ascorbate, flavoring, garlic powder, sodium nitrate, BHA, BHT, citric acid]), sugar, modified food starch, salt, spices, maltodextrin, hydrolyzed soy protein, hydrolyzed corn protein, paprika, garlic, onion.

French Onion Rings

Onion rings are one of those foods that have been maligned by mass production. That's because you think of onion rings as coming out of deep-fat, trans-fat fryers. But French onion soup uses the very same ingredients: onions, oil, and flour. With this recipe, the onion rings turn out to be very good for you. So if anyone asks, just tell them you're having *French* onion rings!

Time to the Table: 15 minutes ✤ *Serves 6 to 8*

Tricks of the Trade

Make sure that you don't put too many onions in the pan at the same time. The oil should completely surround the onions as they cook.

YOU'LL NEED

Vegetable oil
2 large onions
2 cups all-purpose flour
Salt and freshly ground pepper to taste

IN YOUR PAN

In a large iron skillet, pour in enough oil to be able to just cover your onion rings. Heat the oil over medium-high heat until it's very hot but not smoking.

WHILE THE OIL'S HEATING

Cut the onions transversely so that they separate into little rings.

Put the flour in a Ziploc bag, followed by the onions. Gently move the onions around in the bag to completely cover them with flour, and then place them in the vegetable oil, in batches if necessary, to sauté until golden brown. Remove to a paper towel, season with salt and pepper, and eat immediately.

Play with Your Food

To spice up your rings, you can throw any of your favorite spices into the bag with the flour to coat your onions with them. Try chili powder or plain cayenne pepper. You might also try your onion rings like the Brits have their fish and chips—with malt vinegar.

FAUX-FOOD EQUIVALENT: *French's Original French Fried Onions*

Ingredients: Partially hydrogenated vegetable oil (soybean and/or cottonseed), wheat flour, onions, soy flour, salt, dextrose, TBHQ and citric acid in propylene glycol.

Your Daily Bread: Baguettes

Before we went to France, we never had bread with every meal. But we returned with the need to feed our fresh bread habit without spending a fortune in specialty stores.

If you have a normal life, you run into a particular problem with making your own bread. Who has time for this when you get home at 5:30 and have to eat sometime before midnight? So I use this basic French bread recipe, but treat it like I would something made in a Crock-Pot. That is, make the time-consuming part in the morning (mix the dough and put it in a bowl in the fridge), let the dough rise while I'm at work, and then finish it up in the evening (form the loaf, cover it, then put it in the oven in one hour). You can also make the dough ball the night before, letting it rise overnight (then form the loaf in the morning and pop it in the oven in the evening).

Time to the Table: 1 day ✤ Makes 2 baguettes

YOU'LL NEED

    1 teaspoon instant yeast

    1¼ cups warm water

    3 cups all-purpose flour

    1½ teaspoons salt

IN A SMALL BOWL

Add the yeast with ¼ cup of the warm water. Let this sit, warm itself, and come alive while you are preparing the rest of the ingredients.

IN A FOOD PROCESSOR OR MIXING BOWL

Combine the flour and salt with the remaining cup of water and mix. Incorporate the yeast into the flour until it forms a slightly sticky ball. Be sure to knead (or process) the dough long enough so that it's smooth when you stretch it by hand (maybe a full minute in a food processor, ten minutes by hand).

Lay the dough out on a board lightly dusted with flour, and knead into a nice round ball. Place the dough into a bowl rubbed with a smear of olive oil, cover with a cloth, and allow the yeast to fluff up the bread until it doubles in volume (at least 1 hour).

Then deflate our enlarged baguette-to-be and form it into 2 long, thin loaves. Cover and allow them to sit and rise again for at least another couple of hours.

Preheat the oven to 450°F. Before putting the loaves in the oven, moisten your hands and rub them over the bread. Then put the loaves in the oven and bake for 30 minutes. When the bread is done, the crust should be firm and the inside light and fluffy. Remove from the oven and allow to cool on a rack for a few minutes.

Play with Your Food

For herbed bread: Try adding a teaspoon of oregano, rosemary, or cumin seeds to the dough in your first mixing. Fresh herbs are even better.

As for the rise time, there is a tradeoff between speed and taste. The natural fermentation that occurs within the loaf as it rises for a longer period of time dramatically adds to the complexity of the flavors you get on the other end. A good way to do this is to give it a "cool rise" by putting it, covered, into the refrigerator overnight.

FAUX-FOOD EQUIVALENT: *Wonder Country White Bread*

Ingredients: Enriched wheat flour (flour, barley malt, ferrous sulfate [iron], niacin, thiamine mononitrate [B1], riboflavin [B2], folic acid), water, high-fructose corn syrup, yeast, soybean oil, salt, calcium sulfate, wheat gluten, soy flour, dough conditioners (may contain: sodium stearoyl lactylate, calcium dioxide, calcium iodate, diammonium phosphate, dicalcium phosphate, monocalcium phosphate, mono- and diglycerides, ethoxylated mono- and diglycerides, calcium).

Somebody's Buttermilk Biscuits

This rich recipe is at least five generations old; I call them *Somebody's* Buttermilk Biscuits because the original source is unknown. Warm up with these on a snowy November morning. Remember that these biscuits go with everything—butter is an obvious first choice, followed closely by milk gravy, sausage gravy (see page 262), tomato gravy, and molasses.

Time to the Table: 20 minutes ✤ *Makes 8 to 12 biscuits*

YOU'LL NEED

    2 cups all-purpose flour
    Pinch of baking soda
    1 teaspoon salt
    3 teaspoons baking powder
    1 tablespoon vegetable oil
    1¼ cups buttermilk
    2 tablespoons unsalted butter

IN A LARGE MIXING BOWL

Mix the dry ingredients (flour, baking soda, salt, and baking powder). Then mix the wet ingredients (oil and buttermilk) into the dry ingredients. You can either stir them around with a wooden spoon, use a food processor, or knead it with your hands until the dough is nice and smooth. If your hands get a bit sticky from the wet dough, just dust a bit of flour on them.

Preheat the oven to 475° F.

ON A CUTTING BOARD

Sprinkle with flour and set the dough on it. Knead it a few times to increase the fluffiness you can expect from the biscuits when they come out of the oven. The dough picks up flour from the board; make sure it takes on just enough to be soft but not sticky.

Form the dough into a round that's about ½ inch thick. Use the open end of a small glass to cut the biscuits.

Dab the glass in flour periodically or it'll get sticky from the wet flour on the inside of the dough. The biscuits you make don't have to be perfectly round, and you can mold them into any shape you want. Put them in a 9-inch baking pan or large iron skillet so they're snug one next to the other. Once they are all sardined in, cut a sliver of butter to place over the top of each.

Bake for about 14 minutes. When you smell them and the tops are golden, take them out and enjoy.

FAUX-FOOD EQUIVALENT: *Pillsbury Hungry Jack Biscuits*

Ingredients: Flour, skim milk, partially hydrogenated soybean oil, sugar, sodium acid pyrophosphate, baking soda, dextrose, salt, vital wheat gluten, water, sodium stearoyl lactylate, mono- and diglycerides, xanthan gum, propylene glycol alginate, calcium sulfate, natural and artificial flavor.

Baked Beans

Baked beans are a commonplace culinary triumph. What began as teeth-splitting flavorless pebbles are transformed by this recipe into pure deliciousness!

Time to the Table: 90 minutes ⚜ *Serves 6 to 8*

YOU'LL NEED

¼ *pound bacon, cut into ½-inch pieces*

2 *tablespoons each of minced onion, celery, and green pepper*

2 *cloves garlic, minced*

2 *15-ounce cans beans, drained*

¼ *cup "Still Kicking" Barbecue Sauce (page 264)*

2 *tablespoons molasses*

2 *tablespoons brown sugar*

continued

1 teaspoon chili powder
1 teaspoon ground cumin
1 teaspoon prepared mustard
1 tablespoon cider vinegar
Splash of Tabasco sauce
Salt and freshly ground pepper to taste

Preheat the oven to 350° F.

IN A FRYING PAN

Fry the bacon until just crisp. Remove the bacon and set aside, and add the onion, celery, green peppers, and garlic to the fat in the pan. Sauté until they are soft and pungent.

TO AN OVEN-SAFE CASSEROLE

Add the beans, vegetables, bacon, and remaining ingredients. Mix until the texture is even. Bake, covered, for 30 minutes. Uncover and bake for 30 minutes more.

Play with Your Food

This recipe is easily adapted to dry beans in the Crock-Pot: Boil 1 pound of rinsed, dried, white beans for 30 minutes. Then drain and add to the Crock-Pot and follow the other instructions above. Put the setting on high and leave all day long, covered.

Substitute spicy Italian sausage for the bacon. You still get the savory addition of the pork, but also enjoy the spice to offset the sweetness of molasses.

FAUX-FOOD EQUIVALENT: *Hanover Baked Beans*

Ingredients: Prepared beans, water, brown sugar, high-fructose corn syrup, sugar, bacon (with water, salt, sugar, sodium phosphate, hydrolyzed soy protein, sodium erythorbate, sodium nitrate), salt, modified corn starch, corn cider vinegar, apple cider vinegar, onion powder, caramel color, spice, natural and artificial color.

Cancer-Fighting Coleslaw

Many foods have properties that safeguard our cells from the rampant reproduction of cancer. One of them is cabbage, which contains the cancer-fighting molecule indole-3-carbinol.

As an added benefit, cabbage is a good source of vitamin C (especially in red cabbage) and folate (especially in Savoy cabbage). This makes it a wonderful staple and an investment in both your short-term and long-term health.

Time to the Table: 15 minutes ✤ Makes enough for 4 servings

Tricks of the Trade

Make sure you slice the cabbage very thin, to maximize the crunch and minimize its chewiness.

The same principle applies to the onions. Just a bit of onion sparks a strong flavor, even for "sweet" onions. These, too, should be finely chopped.

YOU'LL NEED

2 tablespoons mayonnaise
2 teaspoons Dijon or other spicy mustard
Salt and freshly ground pepper to taste
2 cups thinly sliced cabbage
¼ cup finely chopped carrot
¼ cup finely chopped sweet onion

IN A MEDIUM MIXING BOWL

Mix the mayonnaise, mustard, salt, and pepper together. Correct the seasonings, as you like. Mix in the cabbage, carrots, and onion thoroughly. Store in a sealed container in the refrigerator and serve cold.

Play with Your Food

Try adding fruit, such as raisins or apple, or nuts, such as walnuts or pine nuts (these are even better if lightly toasted in a dry pan). To add a bit of acid for balance to this salad, balsamic vinegar is very nice (about 1 to 2 teaspoons).

For those southerners who like their slaw—like their barbecue sauce and baked beans—to have a little sweet twang to it, don't add sugar. Instead, add about 1 to 2 teaspoons cider vinegar and a small clove of garlic, minced.

FAUX-FOOD EQUIVALENT: *Granma's Cole Slaw*

Ingredients: Cabbage, mayonnaise (soybean oil, egg yolks, high-fructose corn syrup, distilled vinegar, mustard [distilled vinegar, mustard seed, salt, spices], water, salt), fructose, sugar, carrots, apple cider vinegar, glucono-delta-lactone, pea fiber, potassium sorbate, salt, erythorbic acid, citric acid, xanthan gum, coloring (water, color [Yellow No. 5, Blue No. 1, propylene glycol, polysorbate 80, turmeric, annatto, potassium hydroxide]).

Perfect Picnic Potato Salad

Look up *picnic* and you'll see a photograph of people sitting around a long wooden table, with a red-and-white-checked tablecloth and a spoon in a large bowl. What's in the bowl? Potato salad. It's the absolute summer must for eating outside. Inexpensive and easy to whip together, this recipe is perfect picnic fare.

Time to the Table: 20 minutes ✤ *Serves 6 to 8*

Tricks of the Trade

Slightly undercook the potatoes so they retain their texture. Remember, too, the smaller the pieces, the faster they'll cook through.

YOU'LL NEED

1½ pounds new potatoes, cubed
½ cup minced parsley

¼ cup minced onion

¼ cup mayonnaise

¼ cup Dijon mustard

1 tablespoon balsamic vinegar

Salt and freshly ground pepper to taste

PREPARE THE POTATOES

Place potatoes into a pot of boiling salted water. Cook for about 10 minutes, or until the potatoes are almost done.

IN A LARGE BOWL

Mix together the parsley, onion, mayonnaise, mustard, vinegar, salt, and pepper. After the potatoes are done, drain and add them to the bowl. Toss well. Correct the seasonings and serve.

Play with Your Food

For a Mediterranean flavor, try adding capers or olives with very thinly sliced red onions.

For German potato salad, add a little crumbled bacon and some sliced boiled eggs. Chopped sweet pickles add a nice balance to the mix, and a fresh sweet bell pepper gives a terrific crunch.

Grill your potato pieces, after brushing them with olive oil, for a lovely smoky flavor.

FAUX-FOOD EQUIVALENT: *Grandma's Potato Salad with Egg*

Ingredients: Potatoes, salad dressing (soybean oil, water, high-fructose corn syrup, distilled vinegar, egg yolks, salt, sugar, mustard [distilled vinegar, mustard seed, salt, spice], salt, modified corn starch, dextrose, whey protein concentrate, guar gum, xanthan gum, locust bean gum, sodium alginate, onion powder, mustard flour, spices, coloring [propylene glycol, polysorbate 80, turmeric, annatto, potassium hydroxide]), eggs, onion, celery, red peppers, salt, potassium sorbate, coloring (propylene glycol, polysorbate 80, turmeric, annatto, potassium hydroxide).

Buttermilk Cornbread

Making a pone of cornbread is a quick way to add a piping hot bread accompaniment to your meal. I grew up with this as a normal part of meals, especially those with fried fish.

Time to the Table: 20 minutes ✤ *1 pone*

YOU'LL NEED

⅓ *cup all-purpose flour*
⅔ *cup cornmeal*
1½ *teaspoons baking powder*
1 *pinch baking soda*
1 *teaspoon salt*
¾ *cup buttermilk*
1 *large egg*
2 *tablespoons vegetable oil*

Tricks of the Trade

Don't leave the cornbread batter in the skillet too long before putting it into the oven, as it can burn pretty quickly.

Self-rising cornmeal can work just as well and you don't have to fiddle with the baking powder and salt. But that means you must settle on their ratio of cornmeal to flour. This determines how muffin-like or cornbread-like the corn pone turns out. Experiment with the ratio on your own to find the graininess you prefer in your bread.

Preheat the oven to 475° F.

IN A LARGE MIXING BOWL

Mix the dry ingredients together (flour, cornmeal, baking powder, baking soda, and salt). Add the buttermilk, egg, and 1 tablespoon of the oil. Mix until smooth.

Put the remaining 1 tablespoon of oil in a 6-inch iron skillet and heat over medium-high heat until the oil becomes wavy and hot. Pour in the cornbread batter and allow it to sizzle for about 1 minute.

Bake for 12 to 15 minutes, until golden brown.

Play with Your Food

For spicier cornbread, add between ⅛ and ¼ cup minced jalapeño peppers, the same amount of crumbled bacon, and substitute the drippings for the olive oil (or at least supplement) to add a smokiness to the bread.

For corn muffins, increase the cornmeal to flour ratio up to 1 to 1 and add a tablespoon of sugar. Serve with butter and raspberry jam.

FAUX-FOOD EQUIVALENT: *Boston Market Home Style Meals Cornbread*

Ingredients: Cornbread mix (bleached flour, sugar, cornmeal, partially hydrogenated soybean and/or cottonseed oil, whey, modified corn starch, egg yolk, leavening [sodium aluminum phosphate, baking soda], egg white, salt, wheat starch, mono- and diglycerides, xanthan gum, defatted soy flour), water.

Macaroni and Cheese

If your kids are like most, they turn up their noses for the weirdest reasons—like the color of the cheese sauce. If this is the case, try white Cheddars, or yellow, or a combination. You could even let your children decide which is their "favorite."

Time to the Table: 15 minutes ✤ *Serves 4*

YOU'LL NEED

Pinch of salt
Splash of extra-virgin olive oil
2 cups elbow macaroni
2 tablespoons unsalted butter
2 tablespoons all-purpose flour

continued

½ cup half-and-half
1 bay leaf
Salt and freshly ground pepper to taste
1 cup grated sharp Cheddar cheese, or more to taste

Tricks of the Trade

The only real trick to this is to remove the pasta from the water a bit underdone. It finishes cooking when you add it back to the sauce.

TO A MEDIUM SAUCEPAN

Add 4 cups of water and the salt and olive oil. Bring it to a boil, and then add the pasta and cook for 6 to 7 minutes. The pasta should be almost, but not quite, tender when you strain it.

WHILE THE PASTA'S BOILING

In a second saucepan, melt the butter over medium heat. Add the flour, mix it thoroughly with the butter to form a roux, and allow it to brown only slightly. Pour in the half-and-half, bring to a simmer, and add the bay leaf, salt, and pepper. Let these flavors bubble into each other for a few minutes. Remove the bay leaf and whisk until smooth. Stir in the grated cheese to complete the sauce, and let it simmer until the pasta is done. Correct the seasonings.

Drain the pasta and then throw it into the sauce. Stir over medium heat for about 2 minutes.

Play with Your Food

Try ½ cup Parmesan instead of the Cheddar.

FAUX-FOOD EQUIVALENT: *Kraft Macaroni & Cheese,* the Cheesiest
Ingredients: Macaroni (durum wheat flour, wheat flour, niacin, ferrous sulfate, thiamin mononitrate, riboflavin, folic acid), cheese sauce mix (whey, whey protein concentrate, salt, sodium tripoly phosphate,

citric acid, sodium phosphate, lactic acid, calcium phosphate, Yellow No. 5, Yellow No. 6, enzymes, cheese culture).

Comfort Food au Gratin

On chilly evenings, these au gratin potatoes are the perfect comfort food. Between the potatoes, creamy sauce, and cheese, you just can't beat it.

Time to the Table: 1½ hours ✤ *Serves 8*

YOU'LL NEED
> *2 cups thinly sliced potatoes (any kind)*
> *½ large onion, minced*
> *5 tablespoons unsalted butter*
> *3 tablespoons all-purpose flour*
> *2 cups milk*
> *Pinch of salt*
> *Salt and freshly ground pepper to taste*
> *⅓ cup shredded Swiss cheese*

TO BEGIN

Blanch the sliced potatoes in boiling water for about 5 minutes. While the potatoes are cooking, sauté the onions in 2 tablespoons of the butter in a skillet over medium heat, until they begin to pale but have not yet browned. Drain the potatoes and take the onions off the heat.

Preheat the oven to 350° F.

PREPARE THE SAUCE

Melt the remaining 3 tablespoons of butter in a saucepan. Sprinkle in the flour, incorporating it completely while stirring, and allow it to bubble until lightly browned. Add the milk and salt and whisk the roux into the milk. Heat until it comes to a boil for just a minute and then remove from the heat.

Season with salt and pepper to taste.

FINISH THE DISH

Place the potatoes and onions in a lightly buttered 2-quart casserole dish. Pour the sauce over the potatoes and shift around the dish to make sure the sauce seeps throughout the potatoes. Sprinkle the cheese evenly over the top.

Bake for 50 minutes, until the top is golden and bubbly.

Play with Your Food

Add spicy sausage or ham. If you use Polish sausage, slice the links thinly and set them in the pan to bake with the potatoes. If you use spicy ground Italian sausage, sauté it with the onions before adding it to the potatoes. You don't need to make the sauce if you don't want to. Alternatively, just add an equal volume (a cup and a half) of cream.

FAUX-FOOD EQUIVALENT: *Betty Crocker Au Gratin Potatoes*

Ingredients: Potatoes, corn starch, whey, salt, partially hydrogenated soybean oil, Cheddar cheese, flour, maltodextrin, modified corn starch, dried onion, disodium phosphate, nonfat milk, dried garlic, mono- and diglyccrides, sodium citrate, blue cheese, lactic acid, natural flavor, Yellow Lake No. 5, Yellow Lake No. 6, soy flour, sodium bisulfite.

Pine Nut Parmesan Risotto

If you told someone you made rice, they'd yawn. If you told them you made Parmesan risotto with pine nuts, they'd be *très* impressed with your cooking skills. But risotto is just rice dressed up for dinner. Don't be intimidated by dishes like risotto—they're easy to make.

Time to the Table: 25 minutes ⚜ *Serves 4*

YOU'LL NEED

3 tablespoons unsalted butter
½ onion, minced
1 cup arborio rice

¼ cup dry white wine

2 cups chicken stock, heated

¼ cup pine nuts

½ cup Parmesan cheese

¼ cup chopped parsley

Salt and freshly ground pepper to taste

Tricks of the Trade

The key to this recipe is in the adding of the stock to the rice. Be sure that each liquid addition just covers the grains and then cooks down almost completely before you add the next one. However, wait too long and the rice will burn on the bottom of the pan.

IN A HEAVY-BOTTOMED SAUCEPAN

Heat the butter over medium heat and sauté the onion until it softens (about 4 minutes). Increase the heat to medium high and add the rice. Be sure to turn over the rice so that all the grains are coated in the butter. Stir in the wine and let it cook into the rice for another 2 minutes or so.

FOR THE LIQUID

Add the heated chicken stock to the pan a little at a time. Pour in enough to just cover the rice (about ½ cup), and stir only long enough to be certain that the liquid has come in contact with all the rice. Wait until the stock has cooked down into the rice before adding another batch of the stock. Continue in this manner until all the stock has been absorbed by the rice. This should take about 25 minutes, and the rice should be just barely done.

TO FINISH

Toss with the pine nuts, Parmesan, and parsley. Season with salt and pepper to taste.

Play with Your Food

For mushroom risotto, soak dried porcinis in the warmed stock for about 20 minutes to soften and then add them with the onions. Reserve the mushroom-infused stock to pour on the rice as you build the risotto.

FAUX-FOOD EQUIVALENT: *Knorr Risotto Milanese*

Ingredients: Rice, modified food starch, whey, salt, autolyzed yeast extract, rice flour, dehydrated onions, partially hydrogenated soybean oil, cheese powder (cow's milk, salt, cheese cultures, enzymes, maltodextrin, partially hydrogenated soybean oil, corn syrup solids, disodium phosphate), natural flavors, dextrose, spices and coloring (including turmeric, saffron, and annatto).

Cheesecake with a Cinnamon Port Wine Glaze

Time to the Table: 2½ hours ✦ *Makes 1 cheesecake*

Tricks of the Trade

You can make this cake lighter by separating out the whites from the yolks, beating them into a stiff meringue, and folding them in separately.

FOR THE CRUST YOU'LL NEED

2½ *cups graham cracker crumbs*

3 *teaspoons brown sugar*

1 *teaspoon almond extract*

½ *cup (1 stick) unsalted butter, melted*

FOR THE FILLING YOU'LL NEED

3 *8-ounce packages cream cheese, at room temperature*

4 *large eggs*

1 *cup sugar*

1½ *teaspoons vanilla extract*

¼ *cup heavy cream*

¼ *cup sour cream*

FOR THE GLAZE YOU'LL NEED

1 cup port wine

1 cup sugar

1 cinnamon stick

2 whole cloves

1 tablespoon orange juice

1 cup fresh cranberries

MAKE THE CRUST

Preheat the oven to 350°F.

Mix the graham cracker crumbs, brown sugar, almond extract, and butter until it gathers a meal-like texture. Press into the bottom of a standard pie plate. Bake for 12 minutes. Remove from the oven and reduce the heat to 300°F. Let cool.

MAKE THE FILLING

In a large mixing bowl, with electric beaters, beat the cream cheese until smooth. Beat in the eggs and then the sugar and mix until it is a bit fluffy, 3 to 4 minutes. Add the vanilla, cream, and sour cream, stirring with a wooden spoon.

BAKE THE CAKE

Pour the mixture into the crust and set in the oven on the top rack. Bake for 50 minutes or until the cake is just set (the middle should jiggle just a bit). Cool at least 1 hour.

MAKE THE GLAZE

In a medium saucepan, bring the port wine, sugar, cinnamon stick, cloves, and orange juice to a boil, and then lower the heat and simmer for 15 minutes. Add the cranberries and simmer for 10 more minutes. Ladle lightly over the cheesecake to serve.

Play with Your Food

For lemon cheesecake, add the juice of one lemon to the filling (lemon zest is nice here, too). For chocolate cheesecake, add a handful of bittersweet morsels to the batter. This will provide a chocolate crunch to the cake, but you could also melt the chocolate (2 to 3 ounces bittersweet) so that it is completely infused.

FAUX-FOOD EQUIVALENT: *Jell-O No Bake Real Cheesecake Dessert Filling*

Ingredients: Sugar, dextrose, skim milk, milk protein concentrate, lactose, lactic acid, cultures, hydrogenated coconut oil, modified food starch, corn syrup, partially hydrogenated palm kernel oil, calcium sulfate, disodium phosphate, tetrasodium pyrophosphate, lactic acid, calcium lactate, dipotassium phosphate, salt, mono- and diglycerides, propylene glycol monosterate, hydroxypropyl methylcellulose, sodium caseinate, acetylated monoglycerides, cellulose gel, hydroxylated soy lecithin, artificial and natural flavors, Yellow No. 5, Yellow No. 6, citric acid, and BHA.

Crust mix: Enriched wheat flour, sugar, partially hydrogenated soybean oil, graham flour, honey, high-fructose corn syrup, salt, baking soda, calcium phosphate, artificial flavor, malted barley flour.

Chewy Chocolate Brownies

These fudgy, chewy, gooey brownies, served with a mound of melting ice cream, are a more than adequate replacement for the boxed mix. And do you know how long it takes to put this together? About 15 minutes. Make these brownies tonight, and reserve the scrapings from the mixing bowl for the kids who volunteer to do dishes.

Time to the Table: 50 minutes ✤ *Makes 12 to 15 brownies*

Tricks of the Trade

What you do with your butter will matter to the final brownie product. For a denser, fudgelike brownie, melt the butter beforehand. But for a lighter texture, cream it together with the sugar and eggs.

YOU'LL NEED

> 6 1-ounce squares of semisweet chocolate
> ½ cup (1 stick) unsalted butter, melted
> 2 tablespoons cocoa powder
> 1 teaspoon instant coffee granules
> 1 cup brown sugar
> 3 large eggs
> 2 teaspoons vanilla extract
> ½ teaspoon salt
> 1 cup all-purpose flour
> 1 cup chopped walnuts

Preheat the oven to 350° F.

IN A MEDIUM SAUCEPAN

Warm the chocolate, butter, cocoa, and coffee over medium heat until melted and smooth.

IN A LARGE MIXING BOWL

Using an electric mixer, beat together the brown sugar, eggs, vanilla, and salt. While still beating, pour the warm chocolate mixture over the spinning beaters until all (except that which you snitched) is incorporated. Add the flour and walnuts and beat until smooth. Pour into a 9-inch baking pan, prepared by smearing a bit of butter and then sprinkling on some flour. Just tamp off the excess.

Bake for 35 to 40 minutes, or until the brownies are dry at the edges and just moist in the center and a toothpick inserted into the middle comes out clean.

Play with Your Food

For cakelike brownies, use only four squares chocolate, 2 eggs, and 1¼ cups flour.

FAUX-FOOD EQUIVALENT: *Pillsbury Thick 'n Fudgy Deluxe Brownie Mix*

Ingredients: Sugar, flour, partially hydrogenated vegetable oil (soybean and cottonseed oils), chocolate flavor syrup (sugar, water, high-fructose corn syrup, cocoa processed with alkali, salt, citric acid, potassium sorbate, xanthan gum, artificial and natural flavors), cocoa processed with alkali, salt, modified corn starch, natural and artificial flavor, baking soda, nonfat milk, soy lecithin.

Practically Flourless Chocolate Cake

Time to the Table: 50 minutes ❦ *Yield: One 9-inch cake*

YOU'LL NEED

4 1-ounce blocks of semisweet baking chocolate

3 tablespoons brewed coffee

⅔ cup plus 1 teaspoon sugar

½ cup (1 stick) unsalted butter, melted

3 large eggs, separated

¼ teaspoon almond extract

Sprinkle of salt

½ cup cake flour

Butter and flour a 9-inch cake pan. Set aside and preheat the oven to 375° F.

IN A SMALL SAUCEPAN

Melt the chocolate with the coffee over the lowest heat. They will slowly get cozy with each other as you blend together the cake parts.

IN A LARGE MIXING BOWL

Using an electric mixer, beat ⅔ cup of the sugar into the melted butter. You may need to cordon off a "splash zone" at first for the flying sugar/butter mixture, but they'll settle down after a while when the two have become one. Now add the egg yolks and continue beating.

Once your chocolate and coffee have melted together, fold into the egg/butter/sugar mixture and add the almond extract. For purist chocolate aficionados (and for those without almond extract lying around in the cupboard), you could forego this—although it really goes well with the chocolate.

IN A MEDIUM MIXING BOWL

Using an electric mixer, beat the egg whites and salt on high speed until stiff peaks form. Stir in a few dollops of this meringue into the cake batter with a spoon or spatula. Then add a quarter of the cake flour. Mix together until smooth. Keep doing this until all of the meringue and flour are incorporated.

BAKE THE CAKE

Pour the batter into the pan and bake for 25 minutes. The cake is ready when when the edges are done (a toothpick or fork comes out clean), and the center is almost there, but barely undercooked.

Let cool for about 15 minutes before running a knife around the edges and flipping the cake onto a wire rack.

Play with Your Food

To ice, try Silky English Cream (page 327).

For chocolate icing, melt 2 squares of semisweet chocolate with 2 tablespoons strong coffee and stir until smooth. Then add 3 tablespoons butter, stirring all the while, until incorporated. Cool until it spreads easily.

FAUX-FOOD EQUIVALENT: *Sugar-Free Chocolate Crème Cake*

Ingredients: Hydrogenated starch hydrolysate, whole eggs, flour, modified corn starch, soybean oil, leavening (sodium aluminum phosphate, sodium aluminum sulfate, sodium bicarbonate), wheat gluten, propylene glycol monoesters, mono- and diglycerides, sodium steroyl lactylate, salt, aspartame, corn oil, acesulfame K, natural and artificial flavor, sodium proprionate, wheat gluten, cocoa powder processed with alkali, black raven cocoa, chocolate flavor (corn starch, alcohol, water, glycerine, tricalcium phosphate).

Molasses Gingerbread Cake

We don't normally lump molasses in the healthy category with broccoli, carrots, and spinach, but just one tablespoon of molasses contains 20 percent of your recommended daily allowance of potassium, calcium, and iron. It's a health food!

Time to the Table: 45 minutes ✤ *Makes 2 cakes*

YOU'LL NEED

3¼ *cups all-purpose flour*
3 *tablespoons finely minced fresh ginger*
2½ *teaspoons baking soda*
2 *teaspoons ground cinnamon*
Sprinkle of salt
1 *cup dark molasses*
1 *cup brown sugar*
½ *cup sour cream*
2 *large eggs*
2 *teaspoons vanilla extract*
1 *cup boiling water*
1 *cup (2 sticks) unsalted butter, melted*

Preheat the oven to 350° F.

PREPARE 2 BREAD PANS

Smear a bit of butter around the bottom of them, followed by a small sprinkle of flour. Tamp off the excess flour.

IN 2 MEDIUM MIXING BOWLS

Mix together the dry ingredients (flour, ginger, baking soda, cinnamon, and salt) in the first bowl. Combine the wet ingredients (molasses, brown sugar, sour cream, eggs, vanilla, water, and butter) in the second bowl.

Mix the wet and dry ingredients together until smooth. Pour into the baking pans and bake for about 35 minutes, until a toothpick or fork inserted into the cakes comes out clean.

Play with Your Food

If the taste of molasses is too strong for you, reduce the amount to ½ cup of light molasses.

FAUX-FOOD EQUIVALENT: *Duncan Hines Moist Deluxe Spice Cake*

Ingredients: Sugar, flour, vegetable shortening (partially hydrogenated soybean oil), leavening (baking soda, dicalcium phosphate, sodium aluminum phosphate, monocalcium phosphate), artificial coloring including Yellow No. 5 Lake, artificial flavor, cellulose gum, dextrose, polyglycerol esters, propylene glycol monoesters, salt, spices, wheat starch, xanthan gum.

Cuppa Cuppa Cuppa Apple Cobbler

This recipe is remarkably easy. 1 cup, 1 cup, 1 cup, 1 stick. That's all you have to remember: "cuppa cuppa cuppa."

Time to the Table: 35 minutes ✤ *Serves 6 to 8*

YOU'LL NEED

3 Golden Delicious apples, cored, peeled, and sliced
Juice of ½ lemon
1 tablespoon water
1 teaspoon ground cinnamon
½ teaspoon ground nutmeg
1 tablespoon cornstarch
½ cup (1 stick) unsalted butter
1 cup self-rising flour
1 cup sugar
1 cup milk

Preheat the oven to 400° F.

IN A MEDIUM SAUCEPAN

First warm the apples over medium heat with the lemon juice, water, spices, and cornstarch. Turn the apple slices over, gently, to completely coat and cook—until just soft—for no more than 3 minutes. Remove from the heat.

Tricks of the Trade

My first try at this produced a cobbler that tasted wonderful but didn't look so good because the dough didn't fluff up and completely enclose the fruit. The solution is to press your fruit down into the batter just a bit. Then, when your dough springs up in the oven, it will cover the fruit and brown like it's supposed to.

IN AN OVEN-SAFE CASSEROLE DISH

Add the butter and melt over medium heat. In a large bowl blend the flour, sugar, and milk into a silky-smooth batter. With a rubber spatula, scrape the batter out right into the center of the melted butter. Then add the fruit.

Bake for about 20 minutes. It's done when the top is golden and bubbly around the sides. Serve right out of the casserole with some rich vanilla ice cream and a sprinkle of cinnamon over the top.

Play with Your Food

Apple, peach, cherry, and blackberry cobbler can all be made with ease. Seasonal fruits may come and go, but you can have cobbler anytime. Be careful with the gentler fruits like blackberries. When you're coating them early on, turn them gently so they don't smush.

FAUX-FOOD EQUIVALENT: *Apple Filling*

Ingredients: Sliced apples, water, high-fructose corn syrup, corn syrup, modified food starch, spice, erythorbic acid.

Comstock Cherry Pie Filling: Cherries, corn syrup, modified food starch, erythorbic acid, and artificial color (Red No. 40).

All-American Apple Pie

Because there is so little sugar in this pie, and no artificial ingredients, it's perfectly fine to have a slice for breakfast. Enjoy.

Time to the Table: 90 minutes ✤ *Makes 1 pie*

YOU'LL NEED

1 five-pound bag Granny Smith apples, peeled, cored, and sliced into ½-inch wedges

1 teaspoon ground cinnamon

½ teaspoon ground nutmeg

½ cup sugar

2 tablespoons unsalted butter

2 piecrusts

Preheat the oven to 350° F.

IN A LARGE MIXING BOWL

Add the apples (play with the thickness of the wedges, depending on how chunky you like your pieces) with the cinnamon, nutmeg, and sugar. Thoroughly mix them until all the apple chunks are coated.

IN THE PIE DISH

Lay the first piecrust in the dish, making sure all the edges are covered, and then pour in the apple filling. Press the apples down, smooth them out, lick your fingers, and then dot with a few small pats of butter.

Set the second crust over the top and pinch the edges down or mash them with a fork. Go crazy here, and make whatever decorations you like. Put small vertical slits into the main part of the crust to allow some ventilation.

BEFORE BAKING

Tear off two 4-inch-long strips of aluminum foil. Place them around the edges to prevent them from burning. You will need to pinch the two ends of the aluminum sheets together. Then put your creation into the oven and bake for 30 minutes. Remove the foil and return the pie to the oven for 15 minutes more to brown.

Tricks of the Trade

If making your own crust (and you should), put the crust together first and then make the filling. This really saves on time, because as soon as you finish peeling and doctoring the apples, the crust will be ready to roll out.

Play with Your Food

For Dutch apple pie, add ¼ cup cream to the apples prior to baking. And for Christmas, add cranberries and coarsely chopped walnuts, about 2 tablespoons each.

FAUX-FOOD EQUIVALENT: *Wal-Mart Apple Pie*

Ingredients: Apples, flour, sugar, water, partially hydrogenated soybean oil, partially hydrogenated cottonseed oil, high-fructose corn syrup, sweetened condensed milk, coconut oil, corn syrup, maltodextrin, water, butter, partially hydrogenated vegetable oil, modified food starch, salt, potassium sorbate, disodium phosphate, carrageenan, vanilla, pear juice concentrate, artificial flavors, alpha tocopherol, mono- and diglycerides, caramel color, Red No. 40, annatto, vanillin, margarine (partially hydrogenated soybean and cottonseed oils, water, salt, whey, vegetable mono- and diglycerides, soybean lecithin, sodium benzoate, citric acid, artificial flavor, vitamin A palmitate), modified food starch, white syrup (corn syrup, water, fructose, natural and artificial flavor, salt, potassium sorbate), dough (dextrose, gelatinized wheat starch, salt, baking soda, calcium proprionate, vegetable shortening [partially hydrogenated soybean and cottonseed oils], sodium bisulfite), salt, cinnamon, natural and artificial flavors, natural and artificial flavor enhancer (with propylene glycol and water), sodium proprionate, and potassium sorbate.

Basic Milk Shake

Why are milk shakes considered bad for you? Normal ice cream is made of milk and eggs and often a fruit (such as strawberries), and these are all completely natural. If you had two eggs, a glass of milk, and a few fresh strawberries for breakfast, you'd receive high marks from any nutritionist. It becomes bad for you when served in enormous cups, and when commercial versions are spiked with corn syrup, dextrose, sugar, and high-fructose corn syrup.

You don't have to suffer the portion distortion, sugar overload, or faux ingredients to have a milk shake. And this one actually turns out to be a perfectly healthy dessert.

Time to the Table: 5 minutes ✤ *Serves 1*

Tricks of the Trade

Yes, you can make ice cream yourself, but most of the time you're going to use store-bought. The good varieties, such as Breyers, have legible ingredients.

If you don't have espresso cups, you can use a normal coffee cup filled two-thirds full.

YOU'LL NEED
All-natural ice cream
Milk, to your taste

IN A SMALL (6-OUNCE) CUP
Scoop enough ice cream to fill the cup to the top. Pour in the amount of milk you choose and stir until smooth.

Play with Your Food
Most ice creams favor a little fruit in them, especially blueberries. Try adding some cut strawberries as well.

FAUX-FOOD EQUIVALENT: *Slim-Fast*

Ingredients: Sugar, whey protein concentrate, fructose, soy protein isolate, gum arabic, dairy whey, cellulose gel, nonfat dry milk, guar gum, soy fiber, powdered cellulose, maltodextrin, soybean lecithin, carageenan, cellulose gum, dextrose, xanthan gum, aspartame, modified corn starch, artificial flavors.

Magic Chocolate Ganache

Magic is not magic to those who know the trick. This recipe will teach you how to make a dessert so fabulous your friends and family will just stare at you in amazement. Ganache is a perfect frosting for any cake, as the center for truffles, or as a covering for any fruit or unsalted nuts.

Time to the Table: 15 minutes ✤ *Makes almost 2 cups*

YOU'LL NEED

1½ cups half-and-half

8 ounces semisweet chocolate, coarsely chopped

2 tablespoons unsalted butter

1 teaspoon vanilla extract

Tricks of the Trade

Chocolate will scald if you heat it too quickly. So when you're melting it into the cream and butter, chop the chocolate and heat it slowly.

IN A HEAVY-BOTTOMED SAUCEPAN

Warm the half-and-half over medium heat. Reduce the heat to low, add the chocolate, and stir until completely melted. Fold in the butter and stir until it has melted in. Take the pan off the heat, and add the vanilla.

Chocolate ganache can be stored in the freezer for weeks—as if it's going to last that long.

Play with Your Food

Add wonderful flavorings to this basic ganache, such as Baileys, Chambord, strong coffee, dark rum, mint, or bourbon. Try them one at a time, to see which you like best.

FAUX-FOOD EQUIVALENT: *Hershey's Chocolate Syrup*

Ingredients: Water, sugar, fructose, cocoa, caramel color, xanthan gum, salt, citric acid, potassium sorbate, artificial flavoring, sodium benzoate, acesulfame, potassium, a nonnutritive sweetener [as if sugar and fructose weren't enough], artificial coloring including Red No. 40, sulfur dioxide.

Vanilla Pudding

If you've always resorted to those little powder packets of pudding, this recipe will give you the tools to finally give them up forever.

Time to the Table: 7 minutes ✤ *Serves 4*

Tricks of the Trade

The amount of flour added determines the consistency, which ranges from thin, like a sauce, when there is no flour added, to thick, like pie-filling custard, when there is up to ½ cup flour added.

The flour also helps prevent the eggs from scrambling as you heat them.

YOU'LL NEED

⅓ cup sugar

4 large egg yolks, beaten

1 tablespoon all-purpose flour

2 tablespoons cornstarch

2 cups milk

2 tablespoons unsalted butter

1 teaspoon vanilla extract

IN A MEDIUM MIXING BOWL

Blend the sugar into the yolks, flour, and cornstarch.

IN A MEDIUM SAUCEPAN

Scald the milk. Then add it into the egg-sugar mixture in very thin stream as you stir constantly with a spoon.

AFTER ALL THE LIQUID HAS BEEN ADDED TO THE BOWL

Pour the mixture back into the saucepan used to scald the milk over barely medium heat. Stir the custard for 15 minutes, or until it thickens up, coating the back of a spoon. Stir off the heat to cool, and add in the butter and vanilla. Pour through a fine-mesh strainer into ramekins or small cups, cover with plastic, and place in the refrigerator for at least 1 hour to cool and set.

Play with Your Food

For chocolate pudding, add ⅓ cup cocoa to the egg-sugar mixture and reduce the vanilla by ½ teaspoon. Add a pinch of cinnamon.

For mocha pudding, add 2 full tablespoons of strong brewed coffee to the milk.

FAUX-FOOD EQUIVALENT: *Kroger Vanilla Pudding & Pie Filling*

Ingredients: Sugar, dextrose, corn starch, modified food starch, salt, polysorbate 60, calcium, carrageenan, artificial flavor, corn syrup solids, sodium caseinate, Yellow No. 5, Yellow No. 6.

Chocolate-Coated Fruit

A great surprise to pull out of the refrigerator to finish a romantic dinner for two.

Time to the Table: 10 minutes ❦ *Makes ½ cup of ganache*

Tricks of the Trade

Be careful when turning the fruit over, especially if using delicate berries such as raspberries. They are easily crushed.

YOU'LL NEED

> 3 1-ounce squares semisweet chocolate
> 3 tablespoons heavy cream
> 3 tablespoons dry sherry
> ½ teaspoon vanilla extract
> 1 pinch of salt
> Red fruit of your choosing, such as cherries, strawberries, and
> raspberries

IN A SAUCEPAN

Over medium-low heat, melt the chocolate with the cream, sherry, vanilla, and salt. Allow it to lightly simmer for 5 minutes.

Dip the fruit into the chocolate to coat. Keep the coating light. Remove to a small plate and place in the refrigerator to cool until ready to serve.

Play with Your Food

You can create various textures of ganache by varying the proportions of cream and chocolate. Baileys makes a great flavoring for the ganache, as does cognac or brandy.

FAUX-FOOD EQUIVALENT: *Dolci Frutta Chocolate Coating for Fruit*

Ingredients: Sugar, partially hydrogenated vegetable oil (palm kernel and palm), reduced mineral whey powder, dutched cocoa, nonfat dry milk, lecithin, salt, sorbitan tristerate, and vanillin.

Silky English Cream

Just as a sauce enriches and expands the flavors of your meat dishes, this Silky English Cream is perfect to complement your desserts, particularly chocolate cake (page 316).

Time to the Table: 30 minutes ❖ *Makes about 2 cups*

Tricks of the Trade

There are two things to watch out for here, and both come from the same cause—trying to rush through it.

First, if you pour that hot milk in with the egg mixture too fast, you get egg drop soup. Second, if you try to thicken the sauce too fast, you get egg drop soup, because the yolks will be cooked.

YOU'LL NEED

1¾ cups milk

4 large egg yolks

⅓ cup sugar

3 teaspoons cornstarch

1 tablespoon vanilla extract

IN A SAUCEPAN

Scald the milk and over medium-high heat, and then remove from the stove.

IN A MIXING BOWL

Using an electric mixer, beat the egg yolks into the sugar and cornstarch for a couple of minutes until smooth. Set the beaters to a high speed. Dribble in the milk, right on top of the blender blades to distribute the hot milk so the egg mixture is warmed only slowly. When all of the milk has been added, you should have a thin frothy mixture.

IN A SAUCEPAN

Return the mixture to the stove and heat over low heat, stirring with a wooden spoon. It takes about 10 to 15 minutes before it will start to coat the back of your spoon.

Add the vanilla and serve.

Play with Your Food

You can also try some type of liqueur (orange is very nice here in combination with the vanilla, as is brandy; use 1 teaspoon of each).

FAUX-FOOD EQUIVALENT: *Fox's U-Bet Vanilla Syrup*

Ingredients: High-fructose corn syrup, and/or sugar, water, vanillin artificial flavor, citric acid, preserved with benzoate of soda.

Vanilla Whipped Cream

It's so tempting to reach for the corn syrup and hydrogenated oil slurry known as whipped topping. Until, that is, you see how easy and wonderful this recipe is.

Time to the Table: 5 minutes ✤ *Serves 4*

YOU'LL NEED

1 pint whipping cream

1 teaspoon vanilla extract

1 tablespoon sugar

Tricks of the Trade

Don't beat too long or you'll get butter. Not bad, but definitely not whipped cream. Also, the cream whips better in colder temperatures. So if you're having trouble with the texture in the summer or in a warm kitchen, just set the bowl over ice for a few minutes and then beat until fluffy.

IN A MIXING BOWL

Pour in the cream, vanilla, and sugar.

Mix with an electric beater on high until it fluffs. You'll know it's done when the whipped cream gently clings to the lifted beaters, but you can continue to make a stiffer texture if you like.

Play with Your Food

Many flavors can be added to your whipped cream. Depending on the dessert, try a teaspoon of almond or orange extract. A teaspoon of rum makes for a delicious accent, as does a simple sweetening with jam or a drizzle of maple syrup.

FAUX-FOOD EQUIVALENT: *Cool Whip Topping*

Ingredients: Water, corn syrup, partially hydrogenated vegetable oils, high-fructose corn syrup, sodium caseinate, natural and artificial flavors, xanthan gum, guar gum, polysorbate 60, sorbitan monosterate, beta-carotene for color.

Oatmeal Raisin Cookies

More than 95 percent of households consume cookies, amounting to more than 2 billion cookies per year. So, if you are an average person, that works out to 300 cookies per year. The batch below, however, makes only about 12.

Time to the Table: 30 minutes ✤ *Makes 12 to 15 cookies*

Tricks of the Trade

Don't worry about greasing the sheet in this recipe. Because it has a stick of butter in it, the cookies won't stick.

YOU'LL NEED

> ½ *cup (1 stick) unsalted butter, softened*
> ½ *cup brown sugar*
> *1 large egg*
> *1 teaspoon vanilla extract*
> ¾ *cup all-purpose flour*
> *Pinch, each, of baking soda, cinnamon, and salt*

1 cup rolled oats
½ cup raisins

Preheat the oven to 350° F.

IN A LARGE BOWL
Blend the wet ingredients (butter, brown sugar, egg, and vanilla).

IN ANOTHER BOWL
Mix the dry ingredients (flour, baking soda, cinnamon, salt, oats, and raisins) and then fold them into the wet ingredients.

Dollop the dough, in lumps about the size of a Ping-Pong ball, onto a cookie sheet. Bake for 12 to 15 minutes, until golden. Remove to a rack to cool, and fend off the children.

Play with Your Food
For cakelike cookies, add a bit more flour.

For extra filling, throw in another ½ cup of oats or ½ cup of crushed walnuts.

For chewy cookies, take them out of the oven a few minutes early, while they are still soft.

FAUX-FOOD EQUIVALENT: *Aunt Martha's Oatmeal Cookies*

Ingredients: Flour, brown sugar, partially hydrogenated soybean oil, water whey, soy lecithin, sodium benzoate, citric acid, mono- and diglycerides, artificial flavor, beta-carotene color, vitamin A palmitate, oats, pecans, butterscotch morsels (sugar, partially hygrogenated palm kernel oil, coconut oil, skim whey, natural and artificial flavor, soy lecithin, Yellow No. 5 Lake, Yellow No. 6 Lake, Blue No. 2 Lake), eggs, corn syrup, baking soda, salt, natural and artificial flavor.

A Rogue's Gallery of Faux-Food Additives

This "Rogue's Gallery" glossary walks you through some of the most common of the unpronounceable ingredients we're confronted with in standard grocery stores. What is Acesulfame-K? Silicone dioxide sounds like something used in breast implants, so why do they put it in cake batter to prevent "the tombstone"? Hydrogenated oils are in everything—is this the same stuff that endangers our hearts? And how are they different from the trans fats that are all over the news now?

The list of unhealthful ingredients in foods can lead you to just stop eating altogether. But remember that all food additives are not bad, just as all food products are not bad. So, to clear things up a bit, I'm asking the same three questions of some of the most common ingredients: What is it?, What is it doing in my food?, and What is it doing in my body? That way, you can get some basic understanding of the risks involved in eating them. Another wonderful resource, if you would like more information on these, is the Center for Science in the Public Interest.

How to Use the Rogue's Gallery

At one point, scientific studies out of North Carolina told us that cigarettes were not lethal. At another point, scientific studies told us that the products laden with hydrogenated oil were going to save our lives. The science has corrected itself, as it usually does, but the point to keep in mind is that research can be well done, the results agreed upon by peers, and still be dead wrong. But, if that's right, how are you supposed to know what to believe?

Some people adamantly defend newly invented food chemicals, and insist that there's no evidence they're harmful at all. Other people will use anecdotal evidence to argue just as strongly how horrid those products really are.

Do what you know is good for you, not *what you hope will one day turn out to be* healthy. And if there's any uncertainty about a product, just wait fifty years or so until the science sorts itself out and everyone agrees. Until then, don't eat it, so you won't be one of those people others look at and say, "Ooh. Ouch. Look at that. What a shame."

Where your health is concerned, hope is not a good strategy, and certainly don't believe slick product ads. Do what you know is right. Eat real food, not faux-food chemicals, especially

> *when you know* a carrot won't cause heart valve problems
> *when you know* an onion won't raise your triglycerides
> *when you know* a walnut won't contribute to diabetes.

When in doubt, leave it out.

Acesulfame-K

What is it?

Acesulfame-K is sold commercially as Sunette and Sweet One. The FDA approved it in 1988 to be used in chewing gum, dry mixes for beverages, instant coffee and tea, gelatin desserts, puddings, and nondairy creamers, and to be sold separately in packets. By 1998, it was allowed into a broad array of food products such as soft drinks. This artificial sweetener results from the chemical combination of carbon, nitrogen, oxygen, hydrogen, sulfur, and potassium.

What is it doing in my food?

It's about two hundred times sweeter than sugar. For severe diabetics, and those who tremble before the twelve calories found in a teaspoon of sugar, it fills an important commercial niche. Also, unlike aspartame, it retains its sweetness when heated. That's why you find it in so many baking products.

What is it doing in my body?

The Center for Science in the Public Interest has pointed out that the safety tests of Acesulfame-K, conducted back in the 1970s, were very poorly done. In fact, later studies suggest that this chemical actually produces cancer. Acesulfame-K breaks down into another chemical called acetoacetamide, and only 1 percent to 5 percent solutions of this breakdown product added to the diet for three months caused thyroid tumors in experimental animals. Based on this and other data, the FDA has been repeatedly petitioned to reconsider its safety.

Remember, sugar comes from plants. Unless you're diabetic, don't sweat that teaspoon! It sure beats a dose of acetoacetamide and the possibility of a thyroid tumor.

Aspartame

What is it?

Aspartame is a chemical invented by accident in the late 1960s, and it happens to be 180 to 200 times sweeter than sugar. Aspartame is synthesized from L-phenylalanine and L-aspartic acid.

What is it doing in my food?

Good question. It was approved by the FDA, but was pulled from the market when it was discovered that Searle, the manufacturer, had hid the damaging evidence produced by their product. It was reinstated years later through the political connections of its CEO, Donald Rumsfeld. It's now used as a zero calorie alternative to sugar in dry form, and as one of the most common sweeteners of drinks.

What is it doing in my body?

When it is heated to 87° F, aspartame degrades into formic acid, methanol, and formaldehyde. Clinical effects from aspartame have been said to include dizziness, hallucinations, hives, and headaches. Those with PKU (phenylketonuria), as well as pregnant or lactating mothers, should avoid it. People who are sensitive to MSG may also be sensitive to aspartame.

John Olney recently pointed out in the *Journal of Neuropathology and Experimental Neurology* that "the artificial sweetener aspartame is a promising candidate to explain the recent increase in incidence and degree of malignancy of brain tumors. Evidence potentially implicating aspartame includes an early animal study revealing an exceedingly high incidence of brain tumors in aspartame-fed rats compared to no brain tumors in concurrent controls, and the recent finding that the aspartame molecule has mutagenic potential."

Aspartame elicits rancorous ire from scientists who argue strongly that it's lethal and just as much shouting comes from those who insist that it's completely benign. In any case, all can agree that it's certainly not a food.

BHA and BHT

What are they?

Butylated hydroxyanisole (BHA) and butylated hydroxytoluene (BHT) are phenolic compounds that exist as a waxy solid and are synthesized by the reaction of p-cresol with isobutene.

What are they doing in my food?

These chemicals are added to foods as a preservative to keep fats from going rancid. They're used for the same purpose in cosmetics, rubber products, petroleum products, thermoplastics, and packing materials. On food labels you may read that they are added "to maintain product freshness." Their use, however, is completely unnecessary and can be replaced by safer antioxidants, such as vitamin E, or left out altogether.

What is it doing in my body?

Because it's fat soluble, BHT is stored in your fat tissues for an extended period of time. These two chemicals can also interfere with blood clotting, and the International Agency for Research on Cancer considers them carcinogenic. The scientific data have actually shown that they are cancer-causing additives in some cases and not in others. But Dr. Saito and colleagues reported very clearly in *Anticancer Research* that BHA and BHT produce "great cytotoxicity [generates cancer] and apoptosis induction [causes cell death]."

Disodium Inosinate (aka, disodium inosine-5′-monophosphate)

What is it?

Disodium inosinate is the second cousin of MSG, which is another of the nucleotide family of chemicals. It can be synthesized from animal sources such as fish.

Why is it in my food?

Disodium inosinate is added to food products as a flavor enhancer, like the free glutamic acids of MSG. In fact, this additive would be incredibly expensive to use if it were not employed in combination with MSG itself. As one report emphasized, if you find disodium inosinate in your food, you'll find MSG.

What is it doing in my body?

Closely related to MSG, it carries much of its same baggage (see page 342). And a growing number of consumer groups warn against the consumption of this product. Specifically, it is reported to trigger gout, and it is not permitted in foods for infants.

EDTA

What is it?

Ethylenediamine tetraacetic acid is a synthetic amino acid also known as disodium calcium EDTA, tetrasodium EDTA, and disodium dihydrogen EDTA.

What is it doing in my food?

EDTA is put in foods to sequester minerals, such as iron and copper, and it is used as a preservative in some canned foods, to maintain color, prevent fizz loss in carbonated drinks, and prevent the oxidation of meats. It's put in foods as a way to get out trace metals that may have been left behind in products that have been synthesized by metallic machinery.

Many "alternative medicine" practitioners recommend "oral chelation therapy" by taking EDTA supplements. However, a large number of research studies have failed to back up their claims.

What is it doing in my body?

EDTA binds to metal ions in your body. This can be good or bad, as heavy metals such as manganese and mercury that you might get from tainted fish should be removed. However, normal levels of copper, zinc, and nickel are vital to your health and should not be removed by any method, much less by eating EDTA. This is a case in which consuming a chemical (EDTA) to solve a problem (food processing–induced metals in your food) produces more problems by removing the natural levels of metals that should be in your body.

Gums

What are they?

Alginates, carrageenan, guar, locust bean, xanthan, tamarine, karaya, gum arabic, and other gums are carbohydrate polymers often derived from natural products.

What are they doing in my food?

Gums are added for the textural stabilization of foods such as candy, puddings, yogurts, dressings, and powdered drink mixes. They're put into breads, such as microwave cakes, to manipulate the sponginess and keep them soft longer.

What are they doing in my body?

They are not normally absorbed by the body and, because of this, may prevent the absorption of some vitamins. Most research indicates no relation to cancer, although University of Iowa College of Medicine researcher Dr. Joanne Tobacman recently proposed that carrageenan may actually enter cells and lead to their death. Gums have also been identified as allergens in some people. The point to remember is not whether these gums are derived from natural products, but whether the molecules abstracted from them are safe for you in the long term.

High-Fructose Corn Syrup

What is it?

HFCS is a concentrated sweetener made through a three-stage chemical reaction with alpha-amylase, gluco-amylase, and glucose-isomerase.

What is it doing in my food?

Food manufacturers like it because it's sweeter than sugar, new chemical processing methods make it cheaper than sugar, and it mixes into soft drinks much easier (the leading user of HFCS). It helps extend food's shelf life, prevents freezer burn in frozen dinners, and keeps breads such as hot dog buns soft. Most low-fat foods contain this sweetener as well. From a food manufacturing standpoint, it's very cost effective.

What is it doing in my body?

The USDA reported that the consumption of HFCS increased from zero in 1966 to an incredible 62.6 pounds per person in 2001.

Even though it's marketed as just another sugar, the body does not recognize it as such and it does not clear it from the bloodstream like normal sugar. For this reason, your liver has to process it like any other toxin, and it does so by elevating your triglycerides. HFCS consumption is also associated with a fatty liver, obesity, and diabetes.

Hydrogenated Oil

What is it?

Hydrogenation is a chemical hardening process. Oils are cooked under intense heat (up to 400° F) and high pressure in the presence of a reactive metal catalyst such as nickel, zinc, or copper. To sufficiently derange the normal conformation of the oil molecules, chemists bubble hydrogen gas through the mixture as it combines with the metal for up to eight solid hours.

Compare this process to, say, the production of olive oil. To get olive oil, squeeze olives, and out comes the oil—no pressure-cooking and bubbling hydrogen reactions with metal catalysts.

What is it doing in my food?

Hydrogenated oils were not invented to improve your health or weight. Nor were they created to make the food taste any better. Food industries chemically modify ordinary oils to extend the shelf life of their products. It saves them money. It also makes the oils more like saturated fats. In my thinking, this synthetic process gives food a texture, taste, and shelf life that approaches plastic.

What is it doing in my body?

Margarine, vegetable shortening, processed foods, deep-fried restaurant foods, and many fat-free products rely on hydrogenated oils, which contain the trans fatty acids strongly associated with heart disease. That's why the FDA recently required food companies to list the amount of the trans fatty acids found in every product.

The Harvard School of Public Health recently pointed out that cutting back on trans fatty acids could save your life. Metabolic studies clearly show that trans fats increase your LDL ("bad") cholesterol and decrease your HDL ("good") cholesterol—a deadly combination for your heart.

More bad news. Epidemiological studies have shown that eating foods with trans fats is associated with an increased risk of coronary heart disease. That's why, in their article "Trans Fatty Acids and Coronary Heart Disease: Background and Scientific Review" for the School of Public Health, the Harvard people say that the threat to your life is even greater from these oils than from plain saturated fats. "By our most conservative estimate, replacement of partially hydrogenated fat in the U.S. diet with natural unhydrogenated vegetable oils would prevent approximately 30,000 premature coronary deaths per year, and epidemiologic evidence suggests this number is closer to 100,000 premature deaths annually. These reductions are higher than what could be achieved with realistic reductions in saturated fat intake."

So have a bit of butter on your bread, but skip the fast-food french fries and any processed food product with hydrogenated oil.

Lactic Acid

What is it?

Bacteria live in our guts and produce this acid during the natural fermentation of sugar. It's actually vital to our digestion. Our muscles also make lactic acid, but not as a result of bacterial activity. It's a waste product that occurs when they contract too much, and it eventually causes cramps.

What is it doing in my food?

Lactic acid is put in foods as a preservative and stabilizer for fat-reduced food products, in processed cheese, frozen desserts, and carbonated beverages. It is also added to provide tartness. In common fermented products such as sauerkraut, yogurt, and sourdough bread, natural lactic acid is produced by the starter culture bacteria to prevent the growth of undesirable microorganisms and (in the case of the bread) to give it that signature tartness.

What is it doing in my body?

Lactic acid–producing bacteria have been implicated as potent anticancer agents, particularly for the colon. Moreover, the cultures found in yogurt boost both the intestinal and systemic immune systems. Even better, bread made with natural bacteria starters have been shown to improve glucose tolerance.

Lactic acid bacteria in foods like yogurt definitely aid digestion. But this doesn't mean that adding the lactic acid chemical to food products has the same effect as is produced by microorganisms. The context in which the molecule is delivered matters. In other words, the lactic acid found in soda will not have the same beneficial effect as you will get by eating naturally fermented foods.

MSG and Its Derivatives

What is it?

Monosodium glutamate is the sodium salt of L-glutamate, an amino acid.

What is it doing in my food?

MSG is used as a flavor enhancer. The Center for Science in the Public Interest points out that its use allows food companies to lower the amount of real ingredients (such as chicken) they include in their foods (such as chicken soup).

What is it doing in my body?

Scientists use MSG *as a way to induce obesity in lab animals.* In combination with a high caloric diet, MSG has also been shown to cause oxidative stress in the liver. In people, physical reactions to MSG can include headache, tingling, weakness, stomachache, migraine, nausea, vomiting, diarrhea, tightness of the chest, skin rash, or sensitivity to light, noise, or smells. Despite these issues, the FDA and an independent scientific panel (FASEB) have cleared MSG for public consumption.

Be careful though, because MSG is often found in food products but labeled in other ways: monosodium glutamate, glutamic acid, hydrolyzed vegetable protein, hydrolyzed protein, hydrolyzed plant protein, plant protein extract, sodium caseinate, calcium caseinate, yeast extract, textured protein, autolyzed yeast, hydrolyzed oat flour, corn oil. If you find these ingredients on your food label, you'll also find MSG in the product.

Nitrates and Nitrites

What are they?

The chemical formula for nitrite is NO_2, and for nitrate it's NO_3. These are both forms of nitrogen commonly produced when ammonium is chemically modified by certain bacteria.

What is it doing in my food?

These are used in processed meats to preserve them (nitrates are very toxic to bacteria). They also happen to be useful for the food companies to prevent the red color of meat from naturally changing to brown.

What is it doing in my body?

When nitrates are ingested, the body sends them through a cascade of reactions. They are first converted into nitrites, which then get converted into N-nitrosamines, which cause colorectal cancer in lab animals. Nitrites also change the iron of your hemoglobin into methemoglobin, which cannot transport oxygen well and can cause tissue asphyxia. This poses the greatest threat for infants, and has been linked to "blue baby disease."

Although vegetables also contain nitrites, they do not cause a cancer risk because they are typically co-localized with high concentrations of vitamin C, which prevents the formation of the N-nitrosamines. In fact, some corporations have started adding ascorbic acid or erythorbic acid to bacon to try to inhibit nitrosamine formation.

All these issues are exactly why you hear the recommendations to limit nitrites in your foods—particularly processed meats.

Phosphoric Acid

What is it?

Phosphoric acid can be made in two ways, either by the wet process or the thermal (furnace) process. In the wet process, mined phosphate ore is treated with sulfuric acid and detergents. Otherwise, phosphorus is reheated until it becomes liquid and is burned into a new form, phosphorus pentoxide (P_2O_5). This is mixed with the low concentration phosphoric acid and, after a purification process, stored for further processing. Phosphoric acid is corrosive to concrete, most metals, and fabrics.

What is it doing in my food?

Phosphoric acid is used, not surprisingly, to acidify the flavors of soft drinks, jellies, frozen dairy products, bakery products, candy, and cheese products. It is also used as a sequestrant in hair tonics, nail polishes, and skin fresheners. Oddly enough, it was recently added to the drinking water in Winnipeg—not because the drinking water needed a bit more tang to it, but to fight the problem of lead accumulating along sewer pipes. It seems that lead builds up along the pipes, and phosphoric acid slows its reaction and release into the water.

What is it doing in my body?

Phosphoric acid can siphon off your calcium, so you excrete it from your body. When your body loses calcium, it pulls what it needs from your bones. There is a "brittle bone syndrome" in women that is associated with soda consumption, and it's thought to result from the loss of calcium due to the phosphoric acid found in soda.

Phosphates themselves are vital to your health, especially the mineral phosphorus. In fact, the B vitamins niacin and riboflavin are not even digested in the absence of phosphorus. It is also required for healthy bones, teeth, muscles, and even makes up part of your DNA and RNA. Phosphorus regulates energy metabolism, helps the body absorb glucose, and controls the pH balance throughout the body.

But you don't have to get your phosphates from soft drink additives! Just eat real foods, such as fish, eggs, poultry, beans, and nuts. Nothing special is required, and you don't even have to be vegetarian, vegan, or shop at the health food store. Adults require 700 milligrams per day, so if you had three pancakes in the morning (about 400 milligrams) and one cup of chili with beans for lunch (about 400), you'd have all you needed right there.

Potassium Bromate

What is it?

The chemical formula for potassium bromate is $KBrO_3$.

What is it doing in my food?

Potassium bromate is used to increase the volume of bread and to improve its texture. It is also used in the production of fish paste and fermented drinks. Potassium bromate has been banned in most countries. Only the United States and Japan still allow this chemical in their foods.

What is it doing in my body?

I'm just going to show you what's written, in capital letters, on the Materials Safety Data Sheet for this chemical: *"Danger! May be fatal if swallowed. Harmful if inhaled or absorbed through skin. Causes irritation to skin, eyes, and respiratory tract. May cause kidney damage."* This is admittedly written for the powdered form not already put into foods, but it's still arresting to see, especially when you go on to read that potassium bromate is the standard method of choice to induce renal cancer in laboratory animals.

The food companies still using potassium bromate say that it gets broken down to harmless bromide in the body, but this has definitely not been demonstrated by research, which consistently finds bromate residues in bread products.

Propyl Gallate

What is it?

Also known as gallic acid, propyl ester, and n-propyl gallate, propyl gallate is synthesized by the esterification of gallic acid. A drawback for the food industry is that it is unstable at high temperatures.

What is it doing in my food?

Often used in concert with BHA and BHT to chemically preserve fats and oils. Propyl gallate is commonly found in margarine, lard, cereals, snack foods, and salad dressings.

What is it doing in my body?

Propyl gallate can cause gastric irritation and is not permitted for children due to its link with a blood disorder known as methemoglobinemia.

In a 2004 study published in the journal *Mutation Research*, a Japanese research group stated flat out that "propyl gallate, widely used as an antioxidant in foods, is carcinogenic to mice and rats." The results from other studies have been mixed but, at the very least, the potential for this chemical to cause cancer is clear.

Red No. 40 Dye

What is it?

Red No. 40 is a great name. Can you imagine how large the ingredient list would be if they had to write the real name on all the products that contain this?

2-NAPHTHALENESULFONIC ACID, 6-HYDROXY-5-(2-METHOXY-5-METHYL-4-SULFOPHENYL)AZO), DISODIUM SALT. Whew! The National Academy of Sciences reported that Red No. 40 is the most used colorant with a total daily intake, on average, of 100 milligrams. Yellow No. 5 was a distant second with 43 milligrams. Red No. 40 is derived from coal tar.

What is it doing in my food?

Coloring food is not new. But before the mid-1850s, all dyes were naturally derived. Red No. 40, introduced in the 1960s and approved in the mid-1970s, is now one of only nine colors accepted by the FDA. It reddens our gelatins, puddings, food products, candies, sodas, and the bizarre assortment of ketchup colors.

What is it doing in my body?

Our official food protection agency, the FDA, approved Red No. 40 for this huge daily consumption, but some doctors have suggested that it's not as safe as generally thought. One study in the journal *Toxicology* reported that Red No. 40 reduced reproductive success, resulting in a degree of wasting in offspring brain weight, a general decrease in survival, as well as a decrease in normal vaginal development. It also decreased general activity levels described as "physical and behavioral toxicity" in developing animals. Another study in *Toxicological Science* determined the genotoxicity (read, dangerous to your genes) of several synthetic red tar dyes such as Red No. 40. The result? It's not pretty. DNA damage, particularly in the colon. This, it is now known, can lead to cancer.

Bottom line? We'll probably never be able to find out definitively whether the Red No. 40 in your maraschino cherries contributes to cancer, but the research results suggest that it has that potential.

Silicone Dioxide

What is it?

Sand. No kidding. Silicone dioxide—and this is straight out of the dictionary—occurs "abundantly as quartz, sand, flint, agate, and is used to manufacture a wide variety of materials, notably glass and concrete." Hmm.

What is it doing in my food?

In addition to your food, it's used in foot powder for the same purpose—to prevent clumping. It's called a "flowing agent" because it allows products like boxed cake mix to pour well after a very long time on the shelf. Without silicone dioxide, the mix would eventually pack down and turn into a brick known as the "tombstone." If you don't want a tombstone on your shelf, just refine some sand and toss it in there.

What is it doing in my body?

About thirty years ago now, a World Health Organization (WHO) Expert Committee on Food Additives met and determined that eating sand wasn't bad for you. It doesn't seem to build up in your tissues, and it doesn't get excreted out by your kidneys. This opinion seems to have held up over time, because there has been no more significant work done on this substance in our foods.

Stevia

What is it?

Stevioside. This is a derivative of a natural South American shrub. It is formed from steviol, glucose, and diterpenic carboxylic alcohol.

What is it doing in my food?

Stevioside is about 150 times sweeter than sugar, although it's accompanied by a licorice-like aftertaste. It's not actually in your food yet, because it can't get approval. The FDA, the European Union, and the Canadians have all rejected it.

What is it doing in my body?

Metabolites of stevia (steviol) can reduce fertility in females, and can also result in low birth weight offspring. Incidentally, the indigenous people of Paraguay have used the plant itself as an oral contraceptive.

Steviol has been shown to reduce sperm count in males, and it has the ability to induce mutations of your DNA (Pezzuto, 1985). This compound can also interfere with food metabolism. For these and other reasons, the joint FAO (Food and Agriculture Organization of the United Nations)/WHO Expert Committee on Food Additives has requested further research on stevioside to be submitted by 2007 to determine its safety.

Sulfites (Sulfer Dioxide and Sodium Bisulfite)

What is it?

Sulfur dioxide (SO_2) is produced by reacting sulfur with oxygen by burning sulfur in air (as such, it's a dangerous pollutant). Sodium bisulfite ($NaHSO_3$) is made by dissolving sulfur dioxide in an alkaline solution.

What is it doing in my food?

Sodium bisulfite is used in almost all commercial wines, except for organic wines, as a preservative. You'll also find sulfites used as a preservative in shrimp, frozen potatoes, cookies, pie dough, bottled lemon juice, and dried fruit. In 1986, the FDA banned the use of sulfites on fruits and vegetables that are eaten raw, such as lettuce or apples, as well as on fresh meat and poultry products. They are also used to keep the food looking as if it's not as old as it really is.

What is it doing in my body?

Sulfites can destroy thiamine (that's vitamin B_1), which is critical for nervous system function, normal learning, and digestion. The FDA estimates that 1 percent of people are sensitive to these compounds, although you can develop hypersensitivity to sulfites at any time in your life—and the results can vary from mild to life threatening.

Incidentally, sulfites do not cause red wine headaches. Some people are allergic to sulfites, but this results in flu-like symptoms, not headaches. Red wine headaches are similar to migraines and may be caused by the histamines present in the wine.

TBHQ

What is it?

Tert-butylhydroquinone (TBHQ) is the common acronym for 2-tertiary butyl 1,4 dihydroxy benzene.

What is it doing in my food?

TBHQ is put in our food because it's a very cheap stabilizer for various edible oils and fats. Like so many other chemical additions, this is put into food products in order to extend the shelf life.

What is it doing in my body?

Researchers at St. John's University in New York have now shown the biochemical pathway this molecule can take to produce cancer. Apparently, it can interact with the copper in your body to derange your DNA. This is straight from their report: "Taken together, the above results conclusively demonstrate that the activation of TBHQ by [copper] . . . may participate in oxidative DNA damage in both isolated DNA and intact cells. These reactions may contribute to the carcinogenicity as well as other biochemical activities observed with BHA in animals."

Although prior studies had not found links between cancer and TBHQ alone, the new results show that TBHQ can react synergistically to cause cancers. For example, a Japanese research group recently reported in the journal *Cancer Letters* an interaction between TBHQ and other preservatives, which caused the proliferation of stomach tumors.

Food Sources of Vitamins and Minerals

I n order to get healthful nutrition from food, rather than pills, you have to know where to go for the nutrients you need. Below, you'll find the vitamins and minerals important for your health, along with their most important food sources.

First of all, many people don't understand the difference between the two classes of vitamins: water-soluble and fat-soluble. *Fat-soluble vitamins* (A, D, E, and K) are found (obviously) in fats and oils and tend to be stored in your liver and within fat cells. Some prominent food sources include fish and plant oils. Water-soluble vitamins (C, the B complex group, PABA, and inositol) circulate in the fluid spaces of your body, in the bloodstream, and so can be easily excreted if their concentration gets too high. The only problem with water-soluble vitamins in food is that they can be lost during preparation and processing.

The list below explains each vitamin in three simple categories: *What it is,* which lists the vitamin along with its alternative name in parenthesis; *What it does,* which details the most common health benefits; and *Where you can get it,* which covers the major foods that contain substantial quantities of the vitamin.

Vitamins

What it is	What it does	Where you can get it
Vitamin A (retinol)	Important for good eyesight and the protection of skin and mucous membranes. Involved in the repair of body tissues and resistance to infection. Vitamin A can slow tumor growth, lower cholesterol, and is associated with reduced risk of cancer.	Eggs, butter, sweet potatoes, beef liver, apricots, carrots, cantaloupe, orange squash, peaches, tomatoes, spinach
Vitamin B_1 (thiamine)	Important for proper circulation, muscle tone, appetite regulation, mood stability, fertility, and is associated with the reduction of some cancers.	Molasses, eggs, brewer's yeast, sunflower seeds, Brazil nuts, beef liver, poultry, fish, soybeans, potatoes
Vitamin B_2 (riboflavin)	Important for basic cell metabolism, formation of red blood cells, stress reduction.	Whole grains, almonds, legumes, cheese, fish, molasses, brewer's yeast
Vitamin B_3 (niacin)	Important for normal brain function and memory, circulation, cellular metabolism, and has been associated with reduced cholesterol.	Seafood, liver, chicken, peanuts, brewer's yeast, milk, rhubarb
Vitamin B_5 (pantothenic acid)	Important factor to aid vitamin utilization, energy production, and red blood cell production.	Broccoli, cabbage, eggs, salmon, wheat germ, whole grains, legumes, oranges
Vitamin B_6 (pyridoxine)	Aids immune system function, the metabolism of basic food nutrients, the release of energy stores, and hormone production.	Green leafy veggies, prunes, peas, molasses, legumes, whole-grain rice, most meats
Vitamin B_8 (biotin)	Important for acid-base balance, energy storage, cell growth, basic metabolic function, and is found in skin, bone marrow, and sex organs.	Eggs, legumes, sardines, whole grains
Vitamin B_9 (folic acid)	Vital for production of DNA, amino acids, and red blood cells. Involved in appetite regulation and protein metabolism.	Cheese, dates, cabbage, salmon, asparagus, whole grains, kidney beans, canned tuna, spinach, milk
Vitamin B_{12} (cobalamin)	Aids in the formation of bone marrow, nucleic acids, and red blood cells (and so helps prevent anemia). Vitamin B_{12} is an important part of the immune system and in the regulation of appetite.	Eggs, milk, sardines, canned tuna, cottage cheese

What it is	What it does	Where you can get it
Inositol	Aids in the reduction of cholesterol and the metabolism of fats and cholesterol. It also prevents atherosclerosis, is involved in brain cell nutrition and hair growth, and has been implicated as an anticancer agent.	Molasses, brewer's yeast, grapefruit, oranges, meat, milk, nuts, grains
Vitamin C (ascorbic acid)	One of the most versatile vitamins. Important anticancer agent used in bone, collagen, and red blood cell production; normal healing; in the immune system; for iron absorption; and in cell respiration.	All peppers, citrus fruits, guava, cantaloupe, broccoli, strawberries, kiwi, tomatoes, parsley
Vitamin D (cholecalciferol)	Another potent anticancer agent actually formed from cholesterol. It assists the uptake of calcium; is used in the nervous system; and is important for clot formation, skin respiration; and basic nervous system function	Most canned fish, such as sardines, herring, tuna, and salmon; eggs; butter; and exposure to sunlight
Vitamin E (alpha-tocopherol)	An important antioxidant and fat-soluble vitamin used to protect most body tissues, from muscle fibers to blood vessels. It's involved in normal nervous system function, reproduction, the reduction of cholesterol, and is required for iron absorption. It's also an anticancer agent.	Oils such as soybean, olive, and sunflower; seeds and nuts; whole grains and oats; eggs; tomatoes; beans; peas
Vitamin K (K_1 is phylloquinone, K_2 is menaquinone)	A critical fat-soluble vitamin that is the key factor in blood clotting and the prevention of bruising. It is also important in the prevention of osteoporosis.	Molasses, eggs, fish, tomatoes, yogurt, oatmeal, green leafy veggies, cauliflower

Minerals

Our bodies require at least fourteen minerals to function: sodium, potassium, calcium, phosphorus, magnesium, manganese, fluoride, copper, chromium, iron, iodine, selenium, zinc, and chloride. This table lists each necessary mineral of your diet, and tells you what it is, what it does for you, and where you can get it.

What it is	What it does	Where you can get it
Calcium	Supplies vital structural support for building bones and teeth, making nerves and muscles work, and aids in blood clot formation.	Dairy products, broccoli, tofu, green beans, sardines, almonds, broccoli, and dark leafy veggies
Chloride	Vital for nerve transmission and fluid regulation in cells.	Salt, rye, tomatoes, olives, celery, seaweed
Chromium	Used with the body's blood sugar regulation system to help control the insulin-sugar balance.	Nuts, brewer's yeast, legumes, whole-grain products, most meats, cheese
Copper	A vital part of hemoglobin, it is needed to help iron carry oxygen to all tissues of the body.	Liver, nuts, seafood
Fluoride	Supports teeth by solidifying tooth enamel. It also helps to harden bones.	Sardines, canned salmon, tea, fluoridated drinking water
Iodine	As a part of thyroid hormone, iodine helps regulate the body's energy metabolism.	Table salt, saltwater fish, kelp
Iron	*The* important part of hemoglobin, which brings in oxygen to all tissues of the body.	All meats, spinach, whole grains, artichokes, molasses, nuts, legumes, beans, parsley, green beans, tomato juice, tofu, clams
Magnesium	Like zinc, magnesium is a component of enzymes and it allows them to work properly for energy production, muscle contraction, and bone mineralization, as well as nerve and immune function.	Beans, nuts, legumes, spinach, broccoli, black-eyed peas, cashews, artichokes, navy beans, whole grains
Manganese	Another integral component of a broad variety of enzymes used for basic cellular functions throughout the body.	Strawberries, green leafy veggies, tea, whole grains, pineapple

What it is	What it does	Where you can get it
Phosphorus	Very important for regulating energy metabolism and the acid-base balance. It's also involved in the formation of your cells. Phosphorus is a key element in bones, teeth, and DNA.	Protein-rich foods, nuts, peas, legumes, all meats, eggs, milk
Potassium	Potassium helps keep your blood pressure stable as well as the integrity of your cells. It helps regulate the fluid and electrolyte balance, muscle contractions, and nerve impulse transmission.	Dairy, avocados, bananas, apricots, raisins, canned salmon, chicken, codfish, legumes, beans, spinach, acorn squash, carrots, tomatoes, potatoes, sweet potatoes, molasses
Selenium	Works synergistically with vitamin E to help prevent heart disease and support cell growth. It's also important as an antioxidant by preventing cellular damage by free radicals.	Liver, Brazil nuts, seafood, kidney, butter, eggs, whole grains
Sodium	Maintains fluid and electrolyte balance, relaxes muscles, helps regulate the fluid movements in and out of cells, and is involved in nerve transmission.	Cured meat, soy sauce, bread, milk, canned salmon, cheese, sausage, sauerkraut, tomato juice, tuna
Zinc	Important for cell growth, reproduction, and genetic material. Zinc is a necessary part of three-fourths of all enzymatic activity in the body. It transports vitamin A and helps in wound healing, sperm production, and the normal development of the fetus.	Seafood, beans, nuts, legumes, whole grains, liver, beef, spinach, broccoli, green peas, green beans, tomato juice, turkey (dark meat), lean ham, lean ground beef, yogurt, most cheeses

Selected Bibliography

The Science of the French Approach

Cereda E, Malavazos AE, Favaro C, Pagani AM. "Modified Mediterranean diet and survival: evidence for diet linked longevity is substantial." *British Medical Journal* 330, no. 7503 (June 4, 2005): 1329; author reply 1329–30.

Cristina F. "Mediterrancan diet health benefits may be due to a synergistic combination of phytochemicals and fatty-acids." *BMJ* 331, no. 7508 (July 9, 2005): E366.

Jeffery RW, Utter J. "The changing environment and population obesity in the United States." *Obesity Research* 11 (2003): 12S–22S.

Li Z, Bowerman S, Heber D. "Health ramifications of the obesity epidemic." *Surgical Clinics of North America* 85, no. 4 (August 2005): 681–701.

Rigby NJ, Kumanyika S, James WP. "Confronting the epidemic: the need for global solutions." *Journal of Public Health Policy* 25, nos. 3–4 (2004): 418–34.

Shortt J. "Obesity—a public health dilemma." *Association of peri Operative Registered Nurses Journal* 80, no. 6 (December 2004): 1069–78.

Stein CJ, Colditz GA. "The epidemic of obesity." *Journal of Clinical Endocrinology and Metabolism* 89 (6) (June 2004): 2522–5.

Tessier S, Gerber M. "Comparison between Sardinia and Malta: The Mediterranean diet revisited." *Appetite* no. 45, 2 (October 2005): 121–6.

Trichopoulou A. "Traditional Mediterranean diet and longevity in the elderly: a review." *Public Health Nutrition* 7 (October 7, 2004): 943–7.

Satiety and Brain Mechanisms

Barkeling B, Ekman S, Rossner S. "Eating behavior in obese and normal weight 11-year-old children." *International Journal of Obesity and Related Metabolic Disorders* 16, no. 5 (May 1992): 355–60.

Barkeling B, Rossner S, Sjoberg A. "Methodological studies on single meal food intake characteristics in normal weight and obese men and women." *Int J Obes Relat Metab Disord* 19, no. 4 (April 1995): 284–90.

Elfhag K, Barkeling B, Carlsson AM, Rossner S. "Microstructure of eating behavior associated with Rorschach characteristics in obesity." *Journal of Personality Assessment* 81, no. 1 (August 2003): 40–50.

Esfahani N, Bednar I, Qureshi GA, Sodersten P. "Inhibition of serotonin synthesis attenuates inhibition of ingestive behavior by CCK-8." *Pharmacology Biochemistry and Behavior* 51 (1995): 9–12.

Hoebel BG. "Brain neurotransmitters in food and drug reward." *American Journal of Clinical Nutrition* 42(Suppl) (1985): 1133–1150.

Stacher G, Bauer H, Steinringer H. "Cholecystokinin decreases appetite and activation evoked by stimuli arising from the preparation of a meal in man." *Physiology and Behavior* 23 (1979): 325–331.

Westerterp-Plantenga MS, Smeets A, Lejeune MP. "Sensory and gastrointestinal satiety effects of capsaicin on food intake." *International Journal of Obesity* 6 (June 2005): 682–8.

Drinks

WINE

Bautista MC, Engler MM. "The Mediterranean diet: is it cardioprotective?" *Progress in Cardiovascular Nursing* 20, no. 2 (Spring 2005): 70–6.

Dore S. "Unique properties of polyphenol stilbenes in the brain: more than direct antioxidant actions; gene/protein regulatory activity." *NeuroSignals* 14, nos. 1–2 (2005): 61–70.

Lloyd HM, Rogers PJ. "Mood and cognitive performance improved by a small amount of alcohol given with a lunchtime meal." *Behavior and Pharmacology* nos. 2–3 (June 1997): 188–95.

Pinder RM, Sandler M. "Alcohol, wine and mental health: focus on dementia and stroke." *Journal of Psychopharmacology* 4 (December 2004): 449–56.

Ruf JC. "Overview of epidemiological studies on wine, health and mortality." *Drugs Under Experimental and Clinical Research*, 29 nos. 5–6 (2003): 173–9.

CAFFEINATED BEVERAGES

Armstrong LE. "Caffeine, body fluid–electrolyte balance, and exercise performance." *International Journal of Nutrition and Exercise Metabolism* 12, no. 2 (June 2002): 189–206.

Ilich JZ, Brownbill RA, Tamborini L, Crncevic-Orlic Z. "To drink or not to drink: how are alcohol, caffeine and past smoking related to bone mineral density in elderly women? *Journal of the American College of Nutrition* 21, no. 6 (December 2002): 536–44.

Michels KB, Willett WC, Fuchs CS, Giovannucci E. "Coffee, tea, and caffeine consumption and incidence of colon and rectal cancer." *Journal of the National Cancer Institute* 97, no. 4 (February 16, 2005): 282–92.

Panagiotakos DB, Pitsavos C, Zampelas A, Zeimbekis A, Chrysohoou C, Papademetriou L, Stefanadis C. "The association between coffee consumption and plasma total homocysteine levels: the 'ATTICA' study." *Heart Vessels* 19, no. 6 (November 2004): 280–6.

Raman A, Schoeller DA, Subar AF, Troiano RP, Schatzkin A, Harris T, Bauer D, Bingham SA, Everhart JE, Newman AB, Tylavsky FA. "Water turnover in 458 American adults 40–79 years of age." *American Journal of Physiology—Renal Physiology* 286, no. 2 (February 2004): F394–401.

Ruhl CE, Everhart JE. "Coffee and caffeine consumption reduce the risk of elevated serum alanine aminotransferase activity in the United States." *Gastroenterology* 128, no. 1 (January 2005): 24–32.

Yen WJ, Wang BS, Chang LW, Duh PD. "Antioxidant properties of roasted coffee residues." *Journal of Agricultural and Food Chemistry* 53, no. 7 (April 6, 2005): 2658–63.

WATER

Grandjean AC, Reimers KJ, Bannick KE, and Haven MC. "The effect of caffeinated, non-caffeinated, caloric and non-caloric beverages on hydration." *J Am Coll Nutr* 19 (2000): 591–600.

McKinley MJ, Cairns MJ, Denton DA, Egan G, Mathai ML, Uschakov A, Wade JD, Weisinger RS, Oldfield BJ. "Physiological and pathophysiological influences on thirst." *Physiol Behav* 81, no. 5 (July 2004): 795–803.

Phillips PA, Rolls BJ, Ledingham JG, Morton JJ. "Body fluid changes, thirst and drinking in man during free access to water." *Physiol Behav* 33, no. 3 (September 1984): 357–63.

Valtin H. " 'Drink at least eight glasses of water a day.' Really? Is there scientific evidence for '8 × 8' "? *American Journal of Physiology—Regulatory Integrative and Comparative Physiology* 283, no. 5 (November 2002): R993–1004.

CARBONATED BEVERAGES

French SA, Hannan PJ, Story M. "School soft drink intervention study." *BMJ* 329, no. 7462 (August 14, 2004): E315–16.

Kristensen M, Jensen M, Kudsk J, Henriksen M, Molgaard C. "Short-term effects on bone turnover of replacing milk with cola beverages: a 10-day interventional study in young men." *Osteoporosis International* (May 11, 2005).

Marshall TA, Levy SM, Broffitt B, Warren JJ, Eichenberger-Gilmore JM, Burns TL, Stumbo PJ. "Dental caries and beverage consumption in young children." *Pediatrics* 112, no. 3, pt. 1 (2003): e184–91.

McGartland C, Robson PJ, Murray L, Cran G, Savage MJ, Watkins D, Rooney M, Boreham C. "Carbonated soft drink consumption and bone mineral density in adolescence: the Northern Ireland Young Hearts project." *Journal of Bone and Mineral Research* 18, no. 9 (September 2003): 1563–9.

Murphy M, Hardman, AE. "Training effects of short and long bouts of brisk walking in sedentary women." *Medicine and Science in Sports and Exercise* 30, no. 1 (1998): 152–7.

Schulze MB, Manson JE, Ludwig DS, Colditz GA, Stampfer MJ, Willett WC, Hu FB. "Sugar-sweetened beverages, weight gain, and incidence of type 2 diabetes in young and middle-aged women." *Journal of the American Medical Association* 292, no. 8 (August 25, 2004): 927–34.

Wyshak G, Frisch RE, Albright TE, Albright NL, Schiff I, Witschi J. "Nonalcoholic carbonated beverage consumption and bone fractures among women former college athletes." *Journal of Orthopaedic Research* 7, no. 1 (1989): 91–9.

Distracted Eating

Barkeling B, Linne Y, Melin E, Rooth P. "Vision and eating behavior in obese subjects." *Obesity Research* 11, no. 1 (January 2003): 130–4.

Bellisle F. "Why should we study human food intake behaviour?" *Nutrition Metabolism and Cardiovascular Diseases* 13, no. 4 (August 2003): 189–93.

Boon B, Stroebe W, Schut H, Ijntema R. "Ironic processes in the eating behaviour of restrained eaters." *British Journal of Health Psychology* 7, pt. 1 (February 2002): 1–10.

Dennison BA, Erb TA, Jenkins PL. "Television viewing and television in bedroom associated with overweight risk among low-income preschool children." *Pediatrics* 109, no. 6 (June 2002): 1028–35.

McKinley MJ, Johnson AK. "The physiological regulation of thirst and fluid intake." *News in Physiological Sciences* 19 (February 2004): 1–6.

Saunders R. " 'Grazing': a high-risk behavior." *Obesity Surgery* 14, no. 1 (January 2004): 98–102.

Utter J, Neumark-Sztainer D, Jeffery R, Story M. "Couch potatoes or french fries: are sedentary behaviors associated with body mass index, physical activity, and dietary behaviors among adolescents?" *Journal of the American Dietetic Association* 103, no. 10 (October 2003): 1298–305.

Supplements and Health

Barr SI. "Increased dairy product or calcium intake: Is body weight or composition affected in humans?" *Journal of Nutrition* 133, no. 1 (January 2003): 245S–48S.

Caris-Veyrat C, Amiot MJ, Tyssandier V, Grasselly D, Buret M, Mikolajczak M, Guilland JC, Bouteloup-Demange C, Borel P. "Influence of organic versus conventional agricultural practice on the antioxidant microconstituent content of tomatoes and derived purees; consequences on antioxidant plasma status in humans." *Journal of Agricultural and Food Chemistry* 52, no. 21 (October 20, 2004): 6503–9.

Curhan GC, Willett WC, Speizer FE, Spiegelman D, Stampfer MJ. "Comparison of dietary calcium with supplemental calcium and other nutrients as factors affecting the risk for kidney stones in women." *Annals of Internal Medicine* 126, no. 7 (April 1997): 497–504.

Fontham ETH. "Protective dietary factors and lung cancer." *International Journal of Epidemiology* 19 (1990): S32–S42.

Gaziano JM. "Vitamin E and cardiovascular disease: observational studies." *Annals of the New York Academy of Science* 1031 (December 2004): 280–91.

Goodman GE, Thornquist MD, Balmes J, Cullen MR, Meyskens FL Jr, Omenn GS, Valanis B, Williams JH Jr. "The beta-carotene and retinol efficacy trial: incidence of lung cancer and cardiovascular disease mortality during 6-year follow-up after stopping beta-carotene and retinol supplements." *J Natl Cancer Inst* 96, no. 23 (December 1, 2004): 1743–50.

Koo LC. "Diet and lung cancer 20+ years later: more questions than answers?" *International Journal of Cancer* Suppl10 (1997): 22–9.

Kmietowicz Z. "Food watchdog warns against high doses of vitamins and minerals." *BMJ* 326 (2003): 1001.

Lee DH, Folsom AR, Harnack L, Halliwell B, Jacobs DR Jr. "Does supplemental vitamin C increase cardiovascular disease risk in women with diabetes? *Am J Clin Nutr* 80, no. 5 (November 2004): 1194–200.

Lonn E, Bosch J, Yusuf S, Sheridan P, Pogue J, Arnold JM, Ross C, Arnold A, Sleight P, Probstfield J, Dagenais GR. "Effects of long-term vitamin E supplementation on cardiovascular events and cancer: a randomized controlled trial." *JAMA* 293, no. 11 (March 16, 2005): 1338–47.

Meltzer HM, Haugen M, Alexander J, Pedersen JI. "Vitamin and mineral supplements—required for good health?" *Tidsskrift for Den Norsk Laegenforening* 124, no. 12 (June 17, 2004): 1646–9.

Pan SY, Ugnat AM, Mao Y, Wen SW, Johnson KC. "A case-control study of diet and the risk of ovarian cancer." *Cancer Epidemiology Biomarkers and Prevention* 13, no. 9 (September 2004): 1521–7.

Rock CL, Jacob RA, Bowen PE. "Update on the biological characteristics of the antioxidant micronutrients: vitamin C, vitamin E, and the carotenoids." *J Am Diet Assoc* 96 (1996): 693–702.

Schutte AE, Huisman HW, Oosthuizen W, van Rooyen JM, Jerling JC. "Cardiovascular effects of oral supplementation of vitamin C, E and folic acid in young healthy males." *International Journal for Vitamin and Nutrition Research* 74, no. 4 (July 2004): 285–93.

Sun X, Zemel MB. "Calcium and dairy products inhibit weight and fat regain during ad libitum consumption following energy restriction in Ap2-agouti transgenic mice." *Journal of Nutrition* 134, no. 11 (November 2004): 3054–60.

U.S. Preventive Services Task Force. "Routine vitamin supplementation to prevent cancer and cardiovascular disease." *Nutrition in Clinical Care* 6, no. 3 (October–December 2003): 102–7.

Yochum LA, Folsom AR, Kushi LH. "Intake of antioxidant vitamins and risk of death from stroke in postmenopausal women." *Am J Clin Nutr* 72, no. 2 (August 2000): 476–83.

Zemel MB. "Regulation of adiposity and obesity risk by dietary calcium: mechanisms and implications." *J Am Coll Nutr* 21, no. 2 (April 2002): 146S–151S.

Zemel MB, Miller SL. "Dietary calcium and dairy modulation of adiposity and obesity risk." *Nutrition Reviews* 62, no. 4 (April 2004): 125–31.

Nutrition and Our Food Sources

Agbioworld. GMO (genetically modified organism) foods in the grocery stores: www.agbioworld.org/newsletter_wm/index.php?caseid=archive&newsid=2347.

Camfield PR, Camfield CS, Dooley JM, Gordon K, Jollymore S, Weaver DF. "Aspartame exacerbates EEG spike-wave discharge in children with generalized absence epilepsy: a double-blind controlled study." *Neurology* 42, no. 5 (May 1992): 1000–3.

Caris-Veyrat C, Amiot MJ, Tyssandier V, Grasselly D, Buret M, Mikolajczak M, Guilland JC, Bouteloup-Demange C, Borel P. "Influence of organic versus conventional agricultural practice on the antioxidant microconstituent content of tomatoes and derived purees; consequences on antioxidant plasma status in humans." *J Agric Food Chem* 52, no. 21 (October 20, 2004): 6503–9.

Curl CL, Fenske RA, Elgethun K. "Organophosphorus pesticide exposure of urban and suburban preschool children with organic and conventional diets." *Environmental Health Perspectives* 111, no. 3 (March 2003): 377–82.

Dennis MJ, Burrell A, Mathieson K, Willetts P, Massey RC. "The determination of the flour improver potassium bromate in bread by gas chromatographic and ICP-MS methods." *Food Additives and Contaminants* 11, no. 6 (November–December 1994): 633–9.

Ilich JZ. "A lighter side of calcium: role of calcium and dairy foods in body weight." *Arhiv za Higijenu Rada i Toksikologiju* Mar 56(1) (2005): 33–8.

Lombardi-Boccia G, Lucarini M, Lanzi S, Aguzzi A, Cappelloni M. "Nutrients and antioxidant molecules in yellow plums (*Prunus domestica L.*) from conventional and organic productions: a comparative study." *J Agric Food Chem* 52, no. 1 (January 14, 2004): 90–4.

Magkos F, Arvaniti F, Zampelas A. "Organic food: Nutritious food or food for thought? A review of the evidence." *International Journal of Food Science and Nutrition* 54, no. 5 (September 2003): 357–71.

Parikh SJ, Yanovski JA. *Am J Clin Nutr* "Calcium intake and adiposity." 77, no. 2 (February 2003): 281–7.

de Roos NM, Bots ML, Katan MB. "Replacement of dietary saturated fatty acids by trans fatty acids lowers serum HDL cholesterol and impairs endothelial function in healthy men and women." *Arteriosclerosis Thrombosis and Vascular Biology* 21, no. 7 (July 2001): 1233–7.

Saito M, Sakagami H, Fujisawa S. "Cytotoxicity and apoptosis induction by butylated hydroxyanisole (BHA) and butylated hydroxytoluene (BHT)." *Anticancer Res* 23, no. 6C (November–December 2003): 4693–701.

Tobacman JK, Walters KS. "Carrageenan-induced inclusions in mammary myoepithelial cells." *Cancer Detection and Prevention* 25, no. 6 (2001): 520–6.

Williams CM. "Nutritional quality of organic food: Shades of grey or shades of green?" *Proceedings of the Nutritional Society* 61, no. 1 (February 2002): 19–24.

Worthington V. "Nutritional quality of organic versus conventional fruits, vegetables, and grains." *Journal of Alternative and Complementary Medicine* 7, no. 2 (April 2001): 161–73.

Genes and Obesity

Antonio G, Chiara PA. "A natural diet versus modern Western diets? A new approach to prevent 'well-being syndromes.'" *Digestive Diseases and Sciences* 50(1) (2005): 1–6.

Cutting TM, Fisher JO, Grimm-Thomas K, Birch LL. "Like mother, like daughter: familial patterns of overweight are mediated by mothers' dietary disinhibition." *Am J Clin Nutr* 69, no. 4 (1999): 608–13.

Hill JO, Melanson EL. "Overview of the determinants of overweight and obesity: current evidence and research issues." *Med Sci Sports Exerc* 31, no. 11 Suppl (November 1999): S515–21.

Return to the Family Table

Boutelle KN, Birnbaum AS, Lytle LA, Murray DM, Story M. "Associations between perceived family meal environment and parent intake of fruit, vegetables, and fat." *Journal of Nutrition Education and Behavior* 35, no. 1 (January–February 2003): 24–9.

Eisenberg ME, Olson RE, Neumark-Sztainer D, Story M, Bearinger LH. "Correlations between family meals and psychosocial well-being among adolescents." *Archives of Pediatrics and Adolescent Medicine* 158, no. 8 (August 2004): 792–6.

Gomis-Porqueras P, Peralta-Alva A. "The Macroeconomics of Obesity in the United States" University of Miami, March 28, 2005, http://econwpa.wustl.edu:8089/eps/mac/papers/0503/0503014.pdf.

Hensrud DD. "Diet and obesity." *Current Opinion in Gastroenterology* 20, no. 2 (March 2004): 119–24.

Kobayashi H, Oikawa S, Hirakawa K, Kawanishi S. "Metal-mediated oxidative damage to cellular and isolated DNA by gallic acid, a metabolite of antioxidant propyl gallate." *Mutation Research* 558, nos. 1–2 (March 14, 2004): 111–20.

Neumark-Sztainer D, Hannan PJ, Story M, Croll J, Perry C. "Family meal patterns: associations with sociodemographic characteristics and improved dietary intake among adolescents." *J Am Diet Assoc* 103, no. 3 (March 2003): 317–22.

Neumark-Sztainer D, Wall M, Story M, Fulkerson JA. "Are family meal patterns associated with disordered eating behaviors among adolescents?" *Journal of Adolescent Health* 35, no. 5 (November 2004): 350–9.

Pezzuto JM, Compadre CM, Swanson SM, Nanayakkara NPD, Kinghorn AD. "Metabolically activated steviol, the aglycone of stevioside, is mutagenic." *Proceedings of the National Academy of Sciences* 82, no. 8 (1985): 2478–2482.

Sugar Consumption

Basciano H, Federico L, Adeli K. "Fructose, insulin resistance, and metabolic dyslipidemia." *Nutrition & Metabolism* (Lond) 2, no. 1 (February 21, 2005): 5.

Brand-Miller JC. "Glycemic index in relation to coronary disease." *Asia Pacific Journal of Clinical Nutrition* 13 Suppl (2004): S3.

Davail S, Rideau N, Bernadet MD, Andre JM, Guy G, Hoo-Paris R. "Effects of dietary fructose on liver steatosis in overfed mule ducks." *Hormone and Metabolic Research* 37, no. 1 (January 2005): 32–5.

Krone CA, Ely JT. "Controlling hyperglycemia as an adjunct to cancer therapy." *Integrative Cancer Therapies* 4, no. 1 (March 2005): 25–31.

Rodgers A. "Effect of cola consumption on urinary biochemical and physicochemical risk factors associated with calcium oxalate urolithiasis." *Urological Research* 27, no. 1 (1999): 77–81.

Silvera SA, Jain M, Howe GR, Miller AB, Rohan TE. "Dietary carbohydrates and breast cancer risk: a prospective study of the roles of overall glycemic index and glycemic load." *Int J Cancer* 114, no. 4 (April 20, 2005): 653–8.

Weiss GH, Sluss PM, Linke CA. "Changes in urinary magnesium, citrate, and oxalate levels due to cola consumption." *Urology* 39, no. 4 (April 1992): 331–3.

Portion Size

Diliberti N, Bordi PL, Conklin MT, Roe LS, Rolls BJ. "Increased portion size leads to increased energy intake in a restaurant meal." *Obes Res* 12, no. 3 (March 2004): 562–8.

Kral TV, Roe LS, Rolls BJ. "Combined effects of energy density and portion size on energy intake in women." *Am J Clin Nutr* 79, no. 6 (2004): 962–8.

Levitsky DA, Youn T. "The more food young adults are served, the more they overeat." *J Nutr* 134, no. 10 (October 2004): 2546–9.

Matthiessen J, Fagt S, Biltoft-Jensen A, Beck AM, Ovesen L. "Size makes a difference." *Public Health Nutr* 6, no. 1 (2003): 65–72.

Nielsen SJ, Siega-Riz AM, Popkin BM. "Trends in energy intake in U.S. between 1977 and 1996: similar shifts seen across age groups." *Obes Res* 10, no. 5 (May 2002): 370–8.

Walden HM, Martin CK, Ortego LE, Ryan DH, Williamson DA. "A new dental approach for reducing food intake." *Obes Res* 12, no. 11 (November 2004): 1773–80.

Wansink B, Painter JE, North J. "Bottomless bowls: why visual cues of portion size may influence intake." *Obes Res* 13, no. 1 (January 2005): 93–100.

Young LR, Nestle M. "The contribution of expanding portion sizes to the U.S. obesity epidemic." *Am J Public Health* 92, no. 2 (February 2002): 246–9.

Young LR, Nestle M. "Expanding portion sizes in the U.S. marketplace: implications for nutrition counseling." *J Am Diet Assoc* 103, no. 2 (February 2003): 231–4.

The Effects of Stress

Christie W, Moore C. "The impact of humor on patients with cancer." *Clinical Journal of Oncology Nursing* 9, no. 2 (April 2005): 211–8.

Clark A, Seidler A, Miller M. "Inverse association between sense of humor and coronary heart disease." *International Journal of Cardiology* Aug 80(1) (2001): 87–8.

Fryer S, Waller G, Kroese BS. "Stress, coping, and disturbed eating attitudes in teenage girls." *Int J Eat Disord* 22, no. 4 (December 1997): 427–36.

Parshad O. "Role of yoga in stress management." *West Indian Medical Journal* 53, no. 3 (June 2004): 191–4.

Sassaroli S, Ruggiero GM. "The role of stress in the association between low self-esteem, perfectionism, and worry, and eating disorders." *International Journal of Eating Disorders* 37, no. 2 (March 2005): 135–41.

Index